Handbook of Oral and Maxillofacial Giant Cell Lesions

Kapil Paiwal • Niranzena Panneer Selvam
Abrar Ahmed Alamoudi • Jitin Makker
Anirudha Agnihotry

Handbook of Oral and Maxillofacial Giant Cell Lesions

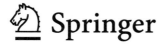

Kapil Paiwal
Oral & Maxillofacial Pathology
Daswani Dental College & Research Center
Kota, Rajasthan, India

Niranzena Panneer Selvam
Oral Health Promotion
Creighton University
Omaha, NE, USA

Abrar Ahmed Alamoudi
Diagnostic Sciences
King Abdul-Aziz University
Jeddah, Saudi Arabia

Jitin Makker
Pathology and Laboratory Medicine
University of California Los Angeles
Los Angeles, CA, USA

Anirudha Agnihotry
Stevenson Dental Research Institute
San Francisco, CA, USA

ISBN 978-981-97-2862-6   ISBN 978-981-97-2863-3   (eBook)
https://doi.org/10.1007/978-981-97-2863-3

© The Editor(s) (if applicable) and The Author(s), under exclusive license to Springer Nature Singapore Pte Ltd. 2024
This work is subject to copyright. All rights are solely and exclusively licensed by the Publisher, whether the whole or part of the material is concerned, specifically the rights of translation, reprinting, reuse of illustrations, recitation, broadcasting, reproduction on microfilms or in any other physical way, and transmission or information storage and retrieval, electronic adaptation, computer software, or by similar or dissimilar methodology now known or hereafter developed.
The use of general descriptive names, registered names, trademarks, service marks, etc. in this publication does not imply, even in the absence of a specific statement, that such names are exempt from the relevant protective laws and regulations and therefore free for general use.
The publisher, the authors and the editors are safe to assume that the advice and information in this book are believed to be true and accurate at the date of publication. Neither the publisher nor the authors or the editors give a warranty, expressed or implied, with respect to the material contained herein or for any errors or omissions that may have been made. The publisher remains neutral with regard to jurisdictional claims in published maps and institutional affiliations.

This Springer imprint is published by the registered company Springer Nature Singapore Pte Ltd.
The registered company address is: 152 Beach Road, #21-01/04 Gateway East, Singapore 189721, Singapore

If disposing of this product, please recycle the paper.

Preface

Welcome to the *Handbook of Oral and Maxillofacial Giant Cell Lesions*. This comprehensive guide is designed to address the complexities and nuances of giant cell lesions within the oral and maxillofacial regions, providing a valuable resource for clinicians, researchers, and students alike.

Giant cell lesions represent a diverse group of conditions characterized by the presence of multinucleated giant cells, and their management requires a nuanced understanding of both clinical presentation and histopathological features. These lesions range from benign to aggressive, and accurate diagnosis is crucial for effective treatment and management.

In this handbook, we delve into the etiology, pathogenesis, and clinical features of these lesions, offering detailed insights into their diagnostic processes. We also explore current therapeutic strategies, ranging from surgical interventions to innovative approaches in medical management. Each chapter integrates up-to-date research and clinical experiences to provide a thorough understanding of these complex conditions.

The aim of this handbook is to equip healthcare professionals with the knowledge and tools necessary to navigate the challenges associated with giant cell lesions. By fostering a deeper understanding of these conditions, we hope to enhance patient outcomes and contribute to the ongoing advancement of oral and maxillofacial care.

I extend my gratitude to the contributing authors and experts who have shared their knowledge and expertise in this field. Their contributions have been instrumental in creating a resource that is both informative and practical.

We trust that this handbook will serve as an invaluable resource in your clinical practice and research endeavors, and we welcome feedback to ensure that it continues to meet the evolving needs of the field.

Sincerely,

Kapil Paiwal

Kota, Rajasthan, India   Kapil Paiwal

Contents

1 Introduction 1

Part I Types of Giant Cells

2 Types of Giant Cells 7

3 Giant Cells in Tumors 9

4 Osteoclast 11

5 Odontoclast 13

Part II Classification of Multinucleated Giant Cells

6 According to Their Occurrence in the Body 17

7 According to Lukas 19

8 According to J. Philip Sapp 21

9 Working Classification of Giant Cell Lesions as Proposed
by Dr. R.V. Subramanyam 23

Part III Lesions

10 Central Giant Cell Granuloma 27

11 Peripheral Giant Cell Granuloma 33

12 Hyperparathyroidism 37

13 Fibrous Dysplasia 43

14 Cherubism 53

15 Paget's Disease 59

16 Giant Cell Tumor of Bone 65

17 Malignant Giant Cell Tumor 67

18 Hodgkin's Disease 71

vii

19	**Aneurysmal Bone Cyst**	75
20	**Calcifying Odontogenic Cyst**	83
21	**Resorption of Teeth**	91
22	**Tuberculosis**	101
23	**Sarcoidosis**	109
24	**Herpes Simplex**	115
25	**Herpes Zoster**	121
26	**Syphilis**	125
27	**Leprosy**	133
28	**Osteomyelitis**	137
29	**Measles**	141
30	**Histoplasmosis**	145
31	**Cryptococcosis**	147
32	**Mucormycosis**	149
33	**Aspergillosis**	153
34	**Wegener's Granulomatosis**	155
35	**Periapical Pathosis**	159
36	**Giant Cell Fibroma**	163
37	**Traumatic Granuloma**	165
38	**Solitary Bone Cyst**	167
39	**Osteoid Osteoma**	171
40	**Osteoblastoma**	175
41	**Radicular Cyst**	179
42	**Cementoblastoma**	185
43	**Osteosarcoma**	189
44	**Actinomycosis**	195
45	**Cat Scratch Disease**	199
46	**Blastomycosis**	203
47	**Rhinosporidiosis**	207

Contents

48 **Giant Cell Arteritis (Temporal Arteritis)** 209

49 **Pyogenic Granuloma**. 211

50 **Pregnancy Epulis or Pregnancy Tumor** 213

Introduction

1

Contents

Reference.. 3

Life began with the appearance of the first cell. The word *cell* comes from the Latin *cella*, meaning "small room." The cell was discovered by Robert Hooke in 1665. He first applied the name cells to the holes that he observed in the cork. He used the word cell because the walls of these holes resembled the walls of a prison cell. In 1835 Jan Evangelista Purkyně observed small "granules" while looking at the plant tissue through a microscope. The cell theory, first developed in 1839 by Matthias Jakob Schleiden and Theodor Schwann, states that all organisms are composed of one or more cells, that all cells come from pre-existing cells, that vital functions of an organism occur within cells, and that all cells contain the hereditary information necessary for regulating cell functions and for transmitting information to the next generation of cells. There are about 10 trillion (10^{13}) cells in human body.

A cell is the basic structural and functional unit of the body and is a biochemical machine. The two principal components of the cell are the cytoplasm, with its multitude of organelles, and the nucleus, with its chromosome and nucleolus. In most cells, the cytoplasm is greater in volume than the nucleoplasm [1]. All cells have a "skin," called the *plasma membrane*, protecting it from the outside environment. The cell membrane regulates the movement of water, nutrients, and wastes into and out of the cell. Inside of the cell membrane are the working parts of the cell. At the center of the cell is the cell *nucleus*. The cell nucleus contains the cell's DNA, the genetic code that coordinates protein synthesis. In addition to the nucleus, there are many *organelles* inside of the cell—small structures that help carry out the

© The Author(s), under exclusive license to Springer Nature Singapore Pte Ltd. 2024
K. Paiwal et al., *Handbook of Oral and Maxillofacial Giant Cell Lesions*, https://doi.org/10.1007/978-981-97-2863-3_1

day-to-day operations of the cell. One important cellular organelle is the *ribosome*. Ribosomes participate in protein synthesis. The transcription phase of protein synthesis takes place in the cell nucleus. After this step is complete, the mRNA leaves the nucleus and travels to the cell's ribosomes, where translation occurs. Another important cellular organelle is the *mitochondrion*. Mitochondria are often referred to as the power plants of the cell because many of the reactions that produce energy take place in mitochondria. Also important in the life of a cell are the *lysosomes*. Lysosomes are organelles that contain enzymes that aid in the digestion of nutrient molecules and other materials.

These cells apart from the inflammatory conditions are also seen in other conditions such as reparative, bacterial, viral, neoplastic, and autoimmune lesions and in lesions due to hormonal imbalance.

The normal cells usually contain a single nucleus with a definitive relationship with the volume of the cytoplasm. But in some situations, the cells might show to contain more than one nucleus sharing a common cytoplasm. The exceptions are the few cells like skeletal muscle cells, cells of placenta, and bone cells which may contain more than one nucleus and are a regular physiological character of these cells. Any other cells exhibiting more than one nucleus or abnormally large-sized nucleus are termed as "giant cells." Such giant cells are significantly found in some conditions such as reactive lesions, chronic inflammatory conditions, and inflammatory granulomatous conditions that characterize these lesions. These conditions along with other several entities, which contain giant cells as predominant findings, are called "giant cell lesions."

Inflammation (Latin, *īnflammō*, "I ignite, set alight") is part of the complex biological response of vascular tissues to harmful stimuli, such as pathogens, damaged cells, or irritants. Inflammation is a protective response intended to eliminate the initial cause of the cell injury as well as the necrotic cells and the tissues resulting from the original insult. It is characterized by an outpouring of leukocytes and plasma into the surrounding tissue.

In case of long-standing infection or chronic inflammation, the lymphocytes derived from the blood become converted into macrophages by the increase in the cytoplasm and enlargement of the nucleus and are involved in the removal of the foreign body particles or the debris. For the same reason, they are also called scavenger cells. When they are unable to deal with the particles or debris to be removed, they fuse together and form multinucleated giant cells which now have the ability to perform their function effectively.

Any of the very large, multinucleated, modified macrophages, which may be formed by coalescence of epithelioid cells or by nuclear division without cytoplasmic division of monocytes, e.g., those characteristics of granulomatous inflammation and those that form around large foreign bodies. Except for the skeletal muscle, placenta, and bone cell, which regularly contain several nuclei, in the same cytoplasm, the occurrence of polykaryons elsewhere in the body is abnormal. The most commonly observed is the inflammatory giant cell (macrophage polykaryon), which appears regularly in response to a wide variety of stimuli. Polykaryons are also seen in many types of tumors and in tissue infected with certain viruses.

The giant cells may contain as many as 50–100 nuclei arranged in various forms within the cytoplasm. The nuclei may be scattered throughout the cytoplasm or arranged either around the periphery in the form of a horseshoe or a ring or may be clustered toward the two poles of the giant cells. The size and the shape of these cells may vary considerably.

Nevertheless, the origin and the mechanism of the formation of multinucleated giant cells remain unclear. It is possible, because of the variety of agents that produce granulomas, that these cells are formed by several different mechanisms. They may arise from the fusion of nonreplicating monocytes or from the mitotic and amitotic division of monocyte nuclei in the absence of cellular division. Several observations suggest that cellular immune mechanisms play a direct role. The giant cells have been found in granulomas of the skin produced by delayed hypersensitivity reactions in humans and in experimental animals.

There is controversy regarding the formation of the multinucleated giant cells in the giant cell granuloma. Adkins suggested that the giant cells are formed by the fusion of the stromal cells, while others support the fact that they originate from endothelial cells of capillaries, fibroblasts, or myofibroblasts.

Reference

1. https://en.wikipedia.org/wiki/Cell_biology#:~:text=Cell%20biology%20(also%20cellular%20biology,living%20and%20functioning%20of%20organisms. Accessed 10 Oct 2023.

Part I
Types of Giant Cells

Types of Giant Cells

2

Contents

2.1   Giant Cells in Inflammation.. 7
     2.1.1   Foreign Body Giant Cells.. 7
     2.1.2   Langhans Giant Cells.. 7
     2.1.3   Touton Giant Cells.. 8
     2.1.4   Aschoff Giant Cells... 8

Various types of giant cells are as follows:

2.1   Giant Cells in Inflammation

2.1.1   Foreign Body Giant Cells

These contain numerous nuclei (up to 100), which are uniform in size and shape and resemble the nuclei of macrophages. These nuclei are scattered throughout the cytoplasm. These are seen in chronic infective granuloma, leprosy, and tuberculosis.

2.1.2   Langhans Giant Cells

Langhans giant cells (also known as Pirogov–Langhans cells) are large cells found in granulomatous conditions. They are formed by the fusion of epithelioid cells (macrophages) and contain nuclei arranged in a horseshoe-shaped pattern in the cell periphery. These were named after Theodor Langhans (1839–1915), a German pathologist.

© The Author(s), under exclusive license to Springer Nature Singapore Pte Ltd. 2024
K. Paiwal et al., *Handbook of Oral and Maxillofacial Giant Cell Lesions*,
https://doi.org/10.1007/978-981-97-2863-3_2

2.1.3 Touton Giant Cells

Touton giant cells are seen in lesions with high lipid content such as fat necrosis, xanthoma, and xanthogranulomas. They are also found in dermatofibroma. They are formed by the fusion of epithelioid cells (macrophages) and contain a ring of nuclei surrounded by a foamy cytoplasm. Touton giant cells are named after Karl Touton. These cells have vacuolated cytoplasm due to lipid content, e.g., in xanthoma.

2.1.4 Aschoff Giant Cells

These multinucleated giant cells are derived from cardiac histiocytes and are seen in the rheumatic nodule.

Giant Cells in Tumors

3

Contents

3.1 Anaplastic Cancer Giant Cells... 9
3.2 Reed–Sternberg Cells.. 9
3.3 Giant Cell Tumor of Bone.. 9

3.1 Anaplastic Cancer Giant Cells

These are larger, have numerous nuclei, which are hyperchromatic, and vary in size and shape. These giant cells are not derived from macrophages but are formed from dividing nuclei of the neoplastic cells, e.g., carcinoma of the liver, various soft tissue sarcomas, etc.

3.2 Reed–Sternberg Cells

These are also malignant tumor giant cells, which are generally binucleated and are seen in various histological types of Hodgkin's lymphoma.

3.3 Giant Cell Tumor of Bone

This tumor of bone has uniform distribution of osteoclast giant cells spread in the stroma.

© The Author(s), under exclusive license to Springer Nature Singapore Pte
Ltd. 2024
K. Paiwal et al., *Handbook of Oral and Maxillofacial Giant Cell Lesions*,
https://doi.org/10.1007/978-981-97-2863-3_3

Osteoclast

4

These multinucleated osteoclasts are much larger cells when compared with all other bone cells and their precursors. Because of their size, they can be identified very easily under light microscope. These are often seen in clusters. Under electron microscope, the cell membrane (adjacent to the tissue surface) is thrown into a myriad of deep folds that form a ruffled border. At the periphery of this border, the plasma membrane is apposed closely to the bone surface; the adjacent cytoplasm is devoid of cell organelles and is enriched in actin, vinculin, and talin proteins (provides integrin-mediated cell adhesion). This clear or ceiling zone not only attaches the cell to the mineralized surface but also isolates a microenvironment between them and the bone surface. Osteoclasts are large multinucleated cells appearing at or near the surface of bone undergoing resorption. They are typically located in cavities or pits (Howship's lacunae) on the bone surface, where it participates in the constant process of bone remodeling.

© The Author(s), under exclusive license to Springer Nature Singapore Pte Ltd. 2024
K. Paiwal et al., *Handbook of Oral and Maxillofacial Giant Cell Lesions*,
https://doi.org/10.1007/978-981-97-2863-3_4

Odontoclast

5

The resorption of dental hard tissue is achieved by cells with a histologic nature similar to that of osteoclast, but because of their involvement in the removal of dental tissue, they are called odontoclasts. Odontoclasts are derived from the monocyte and migrate from blood vessels to the resorption site, where they fuse to form the characteristic multinucleated odontoclast with a clear attachment zone and ruffled border. These are most commonly formed on root surfaces in relation to the advancing permanent tooth; however, they have also been described in the root canals and pulp chamber of resorbing teeth lying against the predentin surface.

These occur singly or in clusters. They are large irregular cells housing up to ten nuclei under electron microscope. These cells have ruffled borders abutting the hard tissue and opposite cell surface bears microvillar processes. The mitochondria and free ribosomes are dense, while r-ER, Golgi apparatus, and vacuoles are moderate.

© The Author(s), under exclusive license to Springer Nature Singapore Pte Ltd. 2024
K. Paiwal et al., *Handbook of Oral and Maxillofacial Giant Cell Lesions,*
https://doi.org/10.1007/978-981-97-2863-3_5

Part II

Classification of Multinucleated Giant Cells

According to Their Occurrence in the Body

6

1. **Physiologic state**
   - (A) Osteoclasts
2. **Pathological state**
   - (A) Damaged striated muscle fibers:
     - Regenerating sarcolemma cells in damaged voluntary muscle
     - Aschoff giant cells in heart muscle (fused myocardial macrophages)
   - (B) Fused fibroblast (giant cell fibroma)
   - (C) Fused macrophages:
     - Due to reaction to foreign bodies (exogenous or endogenous materials), e.g., foreign body giant cells with scattered nuclei
     - Due to reaction to organisms as in tuberculosis and fungal infections, e.g., Langhans giant cell in tuberculosis
     - Touton giant cells of xanthoma
   - (D) Fused cells due to viral infections:
     - Epithelial giant cells as in HSV infections
     - Connective tissue cells as in measles (Warthin–Finkeldey cells)
   - (E) Tumor giant cells:
     - Reed–Sternberg cells in Hodgkin's lymphoma
     - Giant cells in central giant cell granuloma
     - Giant cells in other tumors, e.g., carcinoma

© The Author(s), under exclusive license to Springer Nature Singapore Pte Ltd. 2024
K. Paiwal et al., *Handbook of Oral and Maxillofacial Giant Cell Lesions*,
https://doi.org/10.1007/978-981-97-2863-3_6

According to Lukas

7

1. Intraosseous lesions of the jaw
   (a) The giant cell tumor of bone
   (b) The central giant cell granuloma
   (c) Focal giant cell lesions/brown tumor of hyperparathyroidism
2. Extraosseous lesions
   (a) Giant cell epulis
   (b) Peripheral giant cell granuloma

© The Author(s), under exclusive license to Springer Nature Singapore Pte
Ltd. 2024
K. Paiwal et al., *Handbook of Oral and Maxillofacial Giant Cell Lesions*,
https://doi.org/10.1007/978-981-97-2863-3_7

According to J. Philip Sapp

8

Lesions of the Jaws Containing Giant Cell Tissue

1. Central giant cell granuloma/tumor
2. Peripheral giant cell granuloma
3. Early stage of cherubism
4. Aneurysmal bone cyst
5. "Brown tumor" of hyperparathyroidism

© The Author(s), under exclusive license to Springer Nature Singapore Pte Ltd. 2024
K. Paiwal et al., *Handbook of Oral and Maxillofacial Giant Cell Lesions*,
https://doi.org/10.1007/978-981-97-2863-3_8

Working Classification of Giant Cell Lesions as Proposed by Dr. R.V. Subramanyam

9

1. **Physiological conditions**:
   (a) Resorption of deciduous teeth
   (b) Healing of extraction socket
   (c) Orthodontic tooth movement
2. **Infections**:
   (a) Bacterial: e.g., tuberculosis, syphilis, leprosy, osteomyelitis
   (b) Viral: e.g., herpes simplex, herpes zoster, CMV infection
   (c) Fungal: e.g., histoplasmosis, mucormycosis, aspergillosis, cryptococcosis
   (d) Protozoal: e.g., leishmaniasis
   (e) Chlamydial: lymphogranuloma venereum
3. **Noninfective granuloma**:
   (a) Midline lethal granuloma
   (b) Wegener's granulomatosis
   (c) Plasma cell granuloma
   (d) Sarcoidosis
   (e) Cheilitis granulomatosa
4. **Periodontal conditions**:
   Periodontitis, periapical cyst, periapical granuloma, chronic periapical abscess.
5. **Nonneoplastic growths**:

6. **Cysts and neoplasm**:
   Cyst: aneurysmal bone cyst, calcifying epithelial odontogenic cyst, solitary bone cyst
   Benign neoplasm: giant cell tumor, osteoid osteoma, osteoblastoma, central hemangioma

© The Author(s), under exclusive license to Springer Nature Singapore Pte Ltd. 2024
K. Paiwal et al., *Handbook of Oral and Maxillofacial Giant Cell Lesions*,
https://doi.org/10.1007/978-981-97-2863-3_9

7. **Miscellaneous**:
   (a) Internal resorption
   (b) External resorption
   (c) Massive osteolysis
   (d) Spindle and/or epithelioid cell nevus

A. Soft tissue	B. Bone
– Peripheral giant cell granuloma	– Central giant cell granuloma
– Giant cell fibroma	– Brown tumor of hyperparathyroidism
– Pseudosarcomatous fasciitis	– Fibrous dysplasia
– Epulis fissuratum	– Paget's disease
– Traumatic granuloma	– Cherubism
	– Osteomalacia

Part III

Lesions

Central Giant Cell Granuloma

10

Contents

10.1	Clinical Features	27
10.2	Radiographic Features	28
10.3	Differential Diagnosis	29
10.4	Histopathologic Features	30
10.5	Treatment	31

The giant cell granuloma is considered widely to be a neoplastic lesion. Although formerly designated as "giant cell reparative granuloma," Jaffe gave the term, there is little evidence that the lesion represents reparative response. This entity has various clinical behaviors. Some lesions demonstrate aggressive behavior similar to that of a neoplasm, while others have simple reactive behavior. Most oral and maxillofacial pathologists have dropped the term "reparative." Today these lesions are designated as giant cell granuloma. The World Health Organization defines central giant cell granuloma as an intraosseous lesion consisting of cellular fibrous tissue that contains multiple foci of hemorrhage, aggregations of multinucleated giant cells, and occasionally trabeculae of bone.

10.1 Clinical Features

Central giant cell granulomas may be encountered in patients ranging from 2 to 80 years of age, although more than 60% of all cases occur before age 30. According to Austin, in a study of 34 cases, over 60% of cases occurred before the age of 30 years. Furthermore, 60% of their cases were under the age of 20 years. A majority of giant cell granuloma is noted in females (62–68%). The gender distribution of 38 cases reported by Waldron and Shafer was approximately 2 to 1, females over males. The mandible is the most common site of occurrence of giant cell granu-

© The Author(s), under exclusive license to Springer Nature Singapore Pte Ltd. 2024
K. Paiwal et al., *Handbook of Oral and Maxillofacial Giant Cell Lesions*,
https://doi.org/10.1007/978-981-97-2863-3_10

loma. A majority of lesions appear anterior to the first molar. The giant cell granuloma was originally thought to be peculiar to the jawbones.

Most giant cell lesions are asymptomatic and first to come to attention during routine radiographic examination or as a result of painless expansion of the affected bones. A minority of the cases may be however associated with pain, paresthesia, or perforation of the cortical plate, occasionally resulting in the ulceration of the mucosa by the underlying lesion.

In children, central giant cell granuloma may be responsible for delayed eruption or non-eruption of teeth in the area. Based on the clinical and radiographic features, several groups of investigators have suggested that central giant cell lesions of the jaws may be divided into two categories.

1. Nonaggressive lesions make up most cases, exhibit fewer symptoms, demonstrate slow growth, and do not show cortical perforation or root resorption of teeth involved in the lesion.
2. Aggressive lesions are characterized by pain, rapid growth, cortical perforation, and root resorption. They show a marked tendency to recur after treatment, compared with the nonaggressive type.

10.2 Radiographic Features

Radiographically, central giant cell granulomas present as radiolucent lesions, which may be unilocular or multilocular (Fig. 10.1). Larger lesions are predominantly multilocular (Figs. 10.2 and 10.3). The borders are usually well-defined but poorly corticated. Undulating expansion of the margins may be observed. The classic features of these entities are wispy, faint septa. Some lesions may also have granular bone deposits formed by the entity, giving a mixed appearance. The cortical plates are often thinned and may be perforated by the mass. Displacement and resorption of the teeth are seen with some frequency. In the case of children, the lesions may present with delayed eruption or unerupted teeth.

Whitaker and Waldron (1993) in their study found that 61% of the lesions were multilocular. Most of the cases were well delineated, but 19% had well-corticated borders. Root resorption was evident in 30–43% of cases, while 36% had displaced roots. About 19% of the lesions were associated with impacted or unerupted teeth.

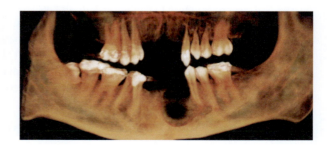

Fig. 10.1 Reconstructed panoramic view with volume rendering showing CGCG lesion in lower anterior area and left mandible. (Courtesy M. Briner, DDS)

10.3 Differential Diagnosis

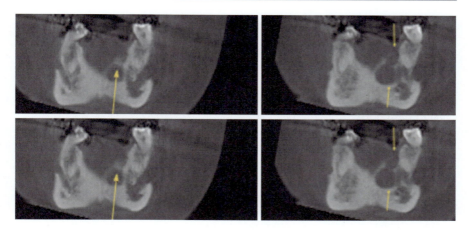

Fig. 10.2 CBCT coronal images of the same patient. Note the wispy septation and the multilocular appearance (yellow arrows)

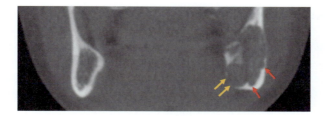

Fig. 10.3 CBCT coronal images of a case of central giant cell granuloma showing a well-defined, non-corticated, radiolucent lesion on the left mandibular region. Note the expansion and thinning of the cortices (orange arrows) and scalloping borders (red arrows)

Advanced imaging such as contrast-enhanced computed tomography (CECT) may be more valuable in the diagnosis of these conditions. With CECT, they are mildly enhancing and soft tissue involvement may be observed. Internal septa emanating at right angles from the cortical border is another classic sign of this lesion. In MRI, they present as hypo–/isointense entities and may be heterogeneously enhanced with contrast.

The radiographic differential diagnosis may include ameloblastoma, odontogenic myxoma, aneurysmal bone cyst, brown tumor of hyperparathyroidism, and cherubism if posterior multifocal lesions are seen.

10.3 Differential Diagnosis

1. **Ameloblastoma**: Occurs usually in older population, located posteriorly in the jaws, with coarse septa and more prominent cortical border.
2. **Brown tumor of hyperparathyroidism**: Occurs in patients with underlying thyroid problem (hyperparathyroidism) and older age group with multiple lesions. Radiological and histopathological findings are similar to CGCG. Any

patient diagnosed with CGCG radiologically and histopathologically should be tested for thyroid function.
3. **Odontogenic myxoma**: Causes less expansion and less root resorption, with characteristic feature of thin and straight septa and lesion border usually scalloped between roots.
4. **Cherubism**: Occurs usually in younger age groups. Lesions are bilateral and start posteriorly.
5. **Aneurysmal bone cyst**: Even though this lesion appears quite similar to CGCG, it is more aggressive and expansile than the latter. CT depicts hypodense vascular spaces within the lesion. T2-weighted MRI may demonstrate fluid–fluid levels.
6. **Hemangioma and arteriovenous malformation**: These lesions may show periosteal reactions and if soft tissue is involved, phleboliths may be seen. If mandible is involved, there could be serpiginous enlargement of the inferior alveolar canal.

10.4 Histopathologic Features

Central giant cell granuloma is made up of a loose fibrillar connective tissue stroma with many interspersed proliferating fibroblasts and small capillaries. Collagen fibers are not usually collected in bundles; however, groups of fibers will often be present. Multinucleated giant cells are prominent throughout the connective tissue, but not necessarily abundant. The giant cells vary in distribution, number, size, shape, and number of nuclei they contain, but they characteristically have distinct eosinophilic or amphophilic cytoplasm (Figs. 10.4 and 10.5).

Whitaker and Waldron (1993) noted that even distributions of the giant cells were found in a large proportion of the recurrent lesions (64%) as opposed to the nonrecurrent lesions (27%).

In addition, there may be foci of old extravasated blood and associated hemosiderin pigment, some of which are phagocytosed by macrophages. Foci of new trabeculae of osteoid or bone also are seen, particularly around the periphery of the lesion. Whitaker and Waldron found that the presence of osteoid within the lesional

Fig. 10.4 Image 4 ×

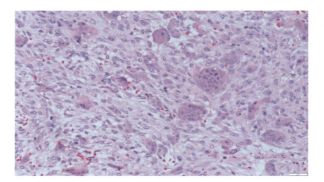

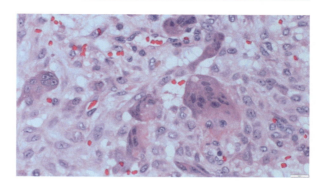

Fig. 10.5 Image 10 ×

tissue was in a larger proportion of the nonrecurrent lesions (56%) as compared with recurrent ones (31%).

10.5 Treatment

Central giant cell lesions of the jaws are usually treated by thorough curettage and enucleation. The recurrence rates range from 11 to 50% or greater. Those lesions, considered on clinical and radiological grounds to be potentially aggressive, show a higher frequency of recurrence. Recurrent lesions often respond to further curettage, although some aggressive lesions require more radical surgery for cure.

In patients with aggressive tumors, three alternatives to surgery, i.e., corticosteroids, calcitonin, and interferon α, are being investigated.

Calcitonin has been found to bind to the calcitonin receptors in the multinucleated giant cells and induces involution and inhibition of DNA synthesis in these cells, thereby reducing their capacity to resorb the bone. Glucocorticoids have also been shown to inhibit the formation of osteoclast-like cells in marrow cultures.

Peripheral Giant Cell Granuloma

11

Contents

11.1	Etiology	33
11.2	Clinical Features	34
11.3	Histopathologic Features	34
11.4	Radiographic Features	35
11.5	Treatment	36
Reference		36

Peripheral giant cell granuloma (PGCG) is a relatively common tumorlike growth of the oral cavity. It probably does not represent a true neoplasm but is a reactive lesion caused by irritation or trauma. Jaffe [1] first suggested the term "giant cell reparative granuloma" for a similar central lesion of the jawbones.

Today, the term "peripheral giant cell granuloma" is universally accepted as the reparative nature of these lesions has not been verified so far. In the past, it was often called as peripheral giant cell reparative granuloma, but the reparative nature appears doubtful.

11.1 Etiology

The etiology of this lesion is not completely understood. However local irritating factors such as tooth extraction, ill-fitting prosthesis, poor restorations, collection of food debris, and calculus seem to play an important role in the development of these lesions.

© The Author(s), under exclusive license to Springer Nature Singapore Pte Ltd. 2024
K. Paiwal et al., *Handbook of Oral and Maxillofacial Giant Cell Lesions*,
https://doi.org/10.1007/978-981-97-2863-3_11

11.2 Clinical Features

Peripheral giant cell granulomas can develop at almost any age but show prevalence in the fifth and sixth decades of life. Approximately 60% of the cases occur in females. The mandible is affected more often than the maxilla, the anterior to molar being the area's most often involved.

The peripheral giant cell granuloma arises from, or is at least attached to, the periodontal ligament or the mucoperiosteum. It occurs exclusively on the gingiva or on the edentulous alveolar ridge, presenting as a pedunculated or sessile red or reddish-blue nodular mass, is vascular or hemorrhagic in appearance, and commonly exhibits surface ulceration.

Peripheral giant cell granuloma is often more bluish-purple when compared with the bright red appearance of the pyogenic granuloma. The lesion varies widely in size but usually is between 0.5 and 1.5 cm in diameter. It can sometimes push the teeth aside and produce "cuffing" resorption of the bone and cause difficulty in determining whether the mass arises as a peripheral lesion or as a central giant cell granuloma that eroded through the cortical bone.

11.3 Histopathologic Features

Microscopically the lesion is unique and consists of nonencapsulated mass of tissue composed of a delicate reticular and fibrillar connective tissue stroma containing large number of ovoid or spindle-shaped young connective tissue cells and multinucleated giant cells; occasionally small amounts of newly formed bone are evident. The giant cells may contain only a few nuclei or up to a dozen (Figs. 11.1 and 11.2). Some of these cells have large vesicular nuclei, whereas others develop small pyknotic nuclei. Abundant hemorrhage is characteristically found throughout the mass, which often results in the deposition of hemosiderin pigment, especially at the periphery of the lesion.

Fig. 11.1 Image 4×

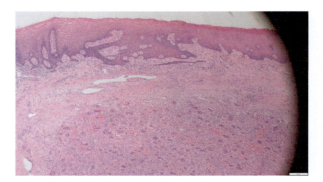

Fig. 11.2 Image 10×

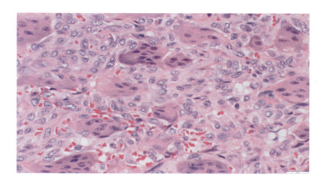

The overlying mucosal surface is ulcerated in about 50% of the cases. A zone of dense fibrous connective tissue usually separates the giant cell proliferation from the mucosal surface. Acute and chronic inflammatory cells are frequently present.

Geschickter and Copeland suggested that the giant cells might be derived from proliferating giant cells associated with the resorption of deciduous tooth roots. So, they suppose the lesion to be concerned with the transition from the deciduous to the permanent dentition.

Another theory of origin is from endothelial cells of capillaries as the occurrence of giant cell within vascular channel suggesting that they arise here through fusion of endothelial cell. Sapp found that these giant cells ultrastructurally contained a sufficient number of features in common with osteoclasts to conclude that they represent a slightly modified form of that cell.

11.4 Radiographic Features

Although the peripheral giant cell granuloma develops within the soft tissue, "cuffing" resorption of the underlying bone is seen in edentulous cases and may show superficial destruction of the interdental bone adjacent to the lesion in dentulous cases (Fig. 11.3). Occasionally it may be sometimes difficult to determine whether the mass arose as a peripheral lesion or as a central giant cell granuloma that eroded through the cortical plate into the gingival soft tissue (Fig. 11.4).

Fig. 11.3 A periapical radiograph showing "cuffing" resorption of the underlying alveolar crest. (Courtesy AZ. Syed, BDS, MHA, MS, Dipl. ABOMR)

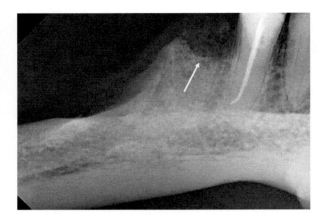

Fig. 11.4 A periapical radiograph of the same patient showing gutta-percha tracing to rule out dental cause

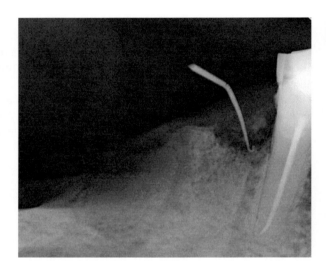

11.5 Treatment

The treatment of the peripheral giant cell granuloma consists of local surgical excision down to the underlying bone. The adjacent teeth should be carefully scaled to remove any source of irritation and minimize the risk of recurrence. Approximately 10% of the lesions are reported to recur and re-excision must be performed.

Reference

1. Jaffe HL. Giant cell reparative granuloma, traumatic bone cyst and fibrous (fibro-osseous) dysplasia of the jawbones. Oral Surg Oral Med Oral Pathol. 1953;6:159–75.

Hyperparathyroidism

12

Contents

12.1	Primary Hyperparathyroidism	37
12.2	Secondary Hyperparathyroidism	38
12.3	Hereditary Hyperparathyroidism	38
12.4	Clinical Features	38
12.5	Radiographic Features	39
12.6	Differential Diagnosis	40
12.7	Histopathologic Features	40
12.8	Diagnosis	40
12.9	Treatment	41

Hyperparathyroidism is produced by the excess production of parathyroid hormone (PTH) which is normally produced by the parathyroid glands in response to a decrease in serum calcium levels. Rarely, it may be associated with a Noonan-type syndrome, a complex, autosomal dominant inherited trait comprising short stature, unusual facies, mental retardation, and cardiac defects. It may be one of the three types—primary, secondary, or hereditary.

12.1 Primary Hyperparathyroidism

Primary hyperparathyroidism (*osteitis fibrosa cystica*) is a condition caused by an overproduction of PTH, in excess of the amount required by the body. It is usually a result of a parathyroid adenoma (80–90% of cases) or parathyroid hyperplasia (10–15% of cases). Infrequently (in less than 2% of cases), a parathyroid carcinoma may be the cause of primary hyperparathyroidism.

Characteristic abnormal findings are elevated parathormone level, calcium and phosphatase levels resulting from parathormone stimulation of osteoclast-mediated

© The Author(s), under exclusive license to Springer Nature Singapore Pte Ltd. 2024
K. Paiwal et al., *Handbook of Oral and Maxillofacial Giant Cell Lesions*, https://doi.org/10.1007/978-981-97-2863-3_12

bone resorption, from decreasing calcium excretion in the kidneys, and from increased intestinal reabsorption. These elevated levels may be manifested by poor muscle tone and decreased muscular excitability.

12.2 Secondary Hyperparathyroidism

It is caused by any condition associated with chronic depression in the serum calcium, because low-level serum calcium leads to compensatory overactivity of parathyroids. It is usually associated with chronic renal disease (patients undergoing renal dialysis) and with intestinal malabsorption syndrome. The mechanism in which the chronic renal insufficiency induces secondary hyperparathyroidism is not fully understood. Chronic renal insufficiency is associated with decreased phosphate excretion, which in turn results in hyperphosphatemia. The elevated serum phosphate levels directly depress serum calcium levels, thereby stimulating parathyroid gland activity. In addition, loss of renal substances reduces the availability of vitamin D, which in turn, reduces intestinal absorption of calcium.

Massry and coworkers reported an incidence of hyperparathyroidism in chronic renal failure patients, ranging from 18% to 92%, after 1 to more than 2 years of dialysis, respectively. Giant cell lesions were not reported until 1963.

12.3 Hereditary Hyperparathyroidism

It is an autosomal dominant condition mapped to chromosome 1q21-q31, the location of the HRPT2 endocrine tumor gene.

12.4 Clinical Features

Hyperparathyroidism is a rare disease which is said to be three times more common in women. It usually occurs in middle age but may occur in childhood or in later life. However in 42 cases, Silverman and his coworkers found no correlation between gender and age and any aspect of the disease. Its incidence increases with age and is greater in postmenopausal women. Early symptoms include fatigue, weakness, nausea, anorexia, arrhythmias, polyuria, thirst, depression, and constipation. Bone pain and headache are often reported.

Patients may have signs and symptoms of hyperparathyroidism and are described as having "stones, bones, abdominal groans and moans."

Stones refer to the fact that these patients, particularly those with primary hyperparathyroidism, have a marked tendency to develop renal calculi (kidney stones, nephrolithiasis) because of the elevated serum calcium levels.

Bones refers to a variety of osseous changes that may occur in conjunction with hyperparathyroidism.

Abdominal groan refers to the tendency for the development of duodenal ulcers.

In addition, moans, i.e., changes in mental status, are often seen, ranging from lethargy and weakness to confusion or dementia.

12.5 Radiographic Features

The bones of affected persons, including the jawbones, show generalized rarefaction manifesting as demineralization and thinning of the cortical borders. Generalized loss of the lamina dura surrounding the roots of the teeth occurs making the teeth stand out in contrast to the surrounding rarefied bone (Fig. 12.1). Alterations in the trabecular pattern may develop. A decrease in trabecular density and blurring of the normal trabecular pattern occur creating a "ground glass" appearance. In the skull, the calvarium may show granular appearance with loss of diploic trabeculae and thinning of the cortical tables. This gives the typical "salt and pepper" appearance.

In long-standing cases, brown tumors may develop in the jaws. They may be solitary or multiple and present the same radiographic features as central giant cell granuloma.

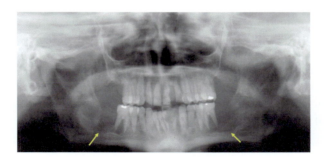

Fig. 12.1 Panoramic radiograph showing bilateral lesions representing brown tumor of hyperparathyroidism in the angle and ramus of the mandible. The lesions are multilocular with non-corticated borders (yellow arrows). Generalized loss of lamina dura and thinning of the mandibular cortices are noted. (Courtesy C. Matesi, DDS)

12.6 Differential Diagnosis

1. **Central giant cell granuloma**: Occurs in the younger population. The lesion is usually located anteriorly in the jaws. Radiological and histopathological findings are similar to brown tumors. Any patient diagnosed with CGCG radiologically and histopathologically should be tested for thyroid function.
2. **Cherubism**: Occurs usually in younger age groups. Lesions are bilateral and start posteriorly.

12.7 Histopathologic Features

The brown tumor of hyperparathyroidism derives its name from the color of the tissue specimen, which is usually a dark reddish-brown because of the abundant hemorrhage and hemosiderin deposition within the tumor.

The most characteristic change in the bone is an osteoclastic resorption of the trabeculae of the spongiosa and along the blood vessels in the Haversian system of cortex. In the areas of resorption, one also finds the plump osteoblasts lining the island of osteoid. Fibrosis of the marrow is marked. In the fibrous islands, there is recent and old hemorrhage, with much hemosiderin being evident. In some instances, collection of osteoclasts, reactive giant cells, and hemorrhagic debris form a distinct mass, termed as "brown tumor of hyperparathyroidism." As the disease progresses, "osteoclastomas" develop, characterized by the masses of fibroblasts growing in a loose syncytium, among which are numerous capillaries and endothelium-lined blood vessels.

Histologic findings in the bone lesions are not pathognomonic of the disease. Laboratory investigations show increased calcium levels that may exceed up to 16–17 mg/dL (normal range 9–12 mg/dL). Some lesions may also show a proliferative response characterized by arrangement of spicules of woven bone set in a cellular fibroblastic background with variable number of multinucleated giant cells. This pattern is often associated with secondary hyperparathyroidism related to chronic renal disease (renal osteodystrophy).

12.8 Diagnosis

It is confirmed by blood investigation which shows hypercalcemia, hypophosphatemia, and elevated serum parathormone level along with hypercalciuria and hyperphosphaturia. The serum alkaline phosphatase level is increased in osteolytic lesions.

12.9 Treatment

For patients with primary HPT and bone disease, such as brown tumor, treatment is directed toward surgical removal of the parathyroid adenomas or three and one half of the hyperplastic glands. The bone lesions tend to resolve spontaneously after correction of the hormonal and metabolic derangement.

Secondary hyperparathyroidism can be controlled by restriction of dietary phosphate, use of phosphate-binding agents, and pharmacologic treatment with an active vitamin D metabolite (e.g., calcitriol). Exposure to aluminum salts, which inhibit bone mineralization, should be eliminated; also patients who do not respond to medical therapy may require parathyroidectomy. Renal transplantation is the ideal treatment because it usually restores the normal physiologic processing of vitamin D, as well as phosphorus and calcium reabsorption and excretion. Patients with multiple tumors should be followed for life. Cinacalcet is a recently approved medical treatment for managing the overproduction of parathormone associated with secondary hyperparathyroidism. This medication is a calcimimetic agent that sensitizes the calcium receptors of the parathyroid cells to extracellular calcium, causing the cells to reduce their output of parathormone.

Fibrous Dysplasia

13

Contents

13.1   Pathology... 44
13.2   Types.. 44
13.3   Monostotic Fibrous Dysplasia.. 45
13.4   Clinical Features.. 45
13.5   Radiographic Features... 45
13.6   Histological Features.. 46
13.7   Polyostotic Fibrous Dysplasia.. 47
13.8   Radiographic Features... 49
13.9   Differential Diagnosis... 50
13.10 Histological Features.. 50
13.11 Oral Manifestations... 51
13.12 Treatment.. 51
References... 51

Fibrous dysplasia is a developmental tumor-like condition of unknown etiology and is characterized by replacement of the normal bone by an excessive proliferation of fibrous connective tissue intermixed with irregular bony trabeculae.

It is a benign fibro-osseous condition involving one or more bones of the cranial and extracranial skeleton consisting of non-encapsulated lesion, which shows replacement of the normal bone by cellular fibrous tissue containing islands of metaplastic bone. Lichtenstein [1] introduced the term fibrous dysplasia. It is thought to be a sporadic condition that results from a post-zygotic mutation in the GNAS I (guanine nucleotide-binding protein, alpha-stimulating activity polypeptide) gene (20q13.2). The gene encodes a G-protein that stimulates the production of c-AMP. The mutation results in a continuous activation of the G-protein leading to overproduction of c-AMP which causes hyperfunction of affected endocrine organs, frequently giving rise to precocious puberty, hyperthyroidism, growth

© The Author(s), under exclusive license to Springer Nature Singapore Pte Ltd. 2024
K. Paiwal et al., *Handbook of Oral and Maxillofacial Giant Cell Lesions*, https://doi.org/10.1007/978-981-97-2863-3_13

hormone, and cortisol overproduction along with increased proliferation of melanocytes resulting in large café-au-lait spots with irregular margins. The clinical severity of the condition depends on the point in time during fetal and postnatal life that the mutation of GNAS 1 occurs.

Clinically fibrous dysplasia may manifest as a localized process involving only one bone or multiple bones or as multiple bone lesions in conjunction with cutaneous and endocrine abnormalities.

If the mutation occurs in one of the undifferentiated stem cells during early embryological life, the osteoblasts, melanocytes, and endocrine cells that represent the progeny of that mutated cell all will carry that mutation and express the mutated gene. The clinical presentation of multiple bone lesions, cutaneous pigmentation, and endocrine disturbances would result. Skeletal progenitor cells at later stages of embryonic development are assumed to migrate and differentiate as part of the process of normal skeletal formation. If the mutation occurs during this later period, the progeny of the mutated cell will disperse and participate in the formation of the skeleton resulting in multiple bone lesions of fibrous dysplasia. Finally, if the mutation occurs during postnatal life, the progeny of that mutated cell is essentially confined to one site, resulting in fibrous dysplasia affecting a single bone.

13.1 Pathology

The skeletal changes have been described by Albright et al. [2], Uehlinger [3], Lichtenstein and Jaffe [4], and Falconer and Cope [5]. Uehlinger stated that the marrow spaces are the site of proliferation of relatively avascular and acellular fibrous tissue which leads to expansion and thinning of the cortex. The long bones and the neighboring bones of the limb girdles are most often affected and the "shepherd's crook" of the femur—a coxa vara deformity—is characteristic. The disease affects primarily the diaphysis: it is exceptional for the epiphyses to be affected. The base of the skull and the bones of the vault are often the site of gross changes which have recently been described by Windholz [6] in a paper in which the relationship between fibrous dysplasia and leontiasis ossea is discussed. No constant changes are found in the blood chemistry other than elevation of the alkaline phosphatase if the bone changes are widespread.

13.2 Types

Clinically fibrous dysplasia can be classified into two main types:

1. Monostotic form involving only one bone, common type
2. Polyostotic forms involving many bones, a less common type, which can be subclassified as:
   (a) Jaffe's type in which several bones of the skeleton are involved

(b) Albright's syndrome, a polyostotic form accompanied by pigmented skin lesions, endocrine dysfunction presenting as precocious puberty in females, and sometimes other anomalies

(c) A craniofacial form confined to bones of the craniofacial complex

(d) Pierce et al. [7] and Zohar et al. [8] described a hereditary craniofacial form of fibrous dysplasia.

13.3 Monostotic Fibrous Dysplasia

This term is applied to those forms of the disease in which only one bone is affected. It occurs in about 70–80% of the cases of FD. It does not manifest extra-skeletal lesions, but may become polyostotic and affect multiple bones. It is less serious than polyostotic form. The clinical term *"leontiasis ossea"* has been applied to cases of monostotic FD which affect maxilla or facial bones and give the patient a leonine appearance.

13.4 Clinical Features

It occurs with equal predilection in males and females with a mild predominance for females. It is more common in children and young adults. Mean age of occurrence is 27–34 years. The maxilla is involved more often than the mandible. Although mandibular lesions are truly monostotic, maxillary lesions often involve adjacent bones, i.e., zygoma, sphenoid, and occiput. The first clinical sign of the disease is a painless swelling or bulging of the jaw. The swelling usually involves buccal plate, labial plate, and seldom the lingual plate. When it involves the mandible, it sometimes causes a protuberant excrescence of the inferior border. The overlying mucosa is almost invariably intact over the lesion. Tenderness may develop. There may be some malalignment, tipping, or displacement of the teeth due to the progressive expansile nature of the lesion. Typical monostotic fibrous dysplasia is characterized by focal poorly circumscribed fibro-osseous replacement of an area of bone.

13.5 Radiographic Features

The radiographic appearance of fibrous dysplasia is extremely variable. The maxilla is twice commonly affected than the mandible, especially the posterior regions more involved. Most of the lesions are unilateral but sometimes may cross the midline in the case of mandible, frontal, and sphenoid bones. The borders are ill-defined, blending with the surrounding normal bone. In younger patients, the lesions may have more well-defined borders. The expansion of the bone is along its long axis maintaining the overall shape. The internal structure may be radiolucent, radiopaque, or a combination of both. This depends mainly on the maturation of the lesion, the early lesions being more radiolucent and the mature lesions more

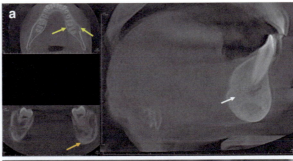
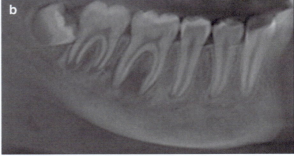

Fig. 13.1 (a) Axial, sagittal, and coronal slices showing bony expansion along the length of the bone (yellow arrow), ground glass internal pattern (white arrows), indistinct inferior border of the mandible (orange arrow) (courtesy N. Shuff, DMD). (b) Cropped custom section of the same patient showing the ground glass internal pattern with no effect on the dentition

radiopaque. The lesions may sometimes have a multilocular pattern. The trabeculae become altered, becoming shorter, thinner, more numerous, irregularly shaped, and randomly oriented. This makes the bone appear more radiopaque. The pattern may resemble any of the following: ground glass, granules orange peel or peau d'orange, finger-/thumbprint, or cotton wool (Fig. 13.1a, b). The heavily ossified lesions may have a pagetoid pattern or a patchy sclerotic appearance. The inferior alveolar canal will be superiorly displaced. The cortical borders of the affected bones and the lamina dura might be indistinct and merge with the altered bone. There might be displacement of teeth. Some of these lesions may develop simple bone cysts or aneurysmal bone cysts.

13.6 Histological Features

The lesion is essentially a fibrous one made up of proliferating fibroblasts in a compact stroma of interlacing collagen fibers (Figs. 13.2 and 13.3).

The trabeculae are thin and located at regular intervals. Irregular trabeculae of bone are scattered throughout the lesion, with no definite pattern of arrangement. Characteristically some of these trabeculae are delicate C-shaped, Chinese character-shaped, or horseshoe-shaped and occasionally may form rings. The trabeculae are usually coarse woven bone but may be lamellar bone. The relationship of osteoblasts and osteoclasts to the trabeculae is similar to that of polyostotic form.

Fig. 13.2 Image 4×

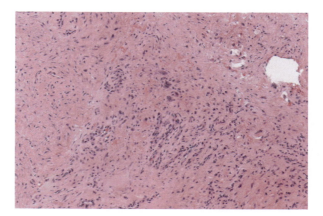

Fig. 13.3 Image 10×

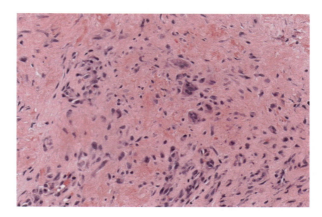

The presence of lamellar bone does not confirm a diagnosis of FD. Other morphological forms of calcification including small rounded bodies (cementum bodies or globular calcifications) as well as minute basophilic and laminated calcification may be seen in FD. The histopathology of FD is not pathognomonic and it should be confirmed by correlation of histopathology, radiography, and clinical features. Giant cells may also be seen in some cases.

13.7 Polyostotic Fibrous Dysplasia

Weil in 1922 recorded the first case of polyostotic fibrous dysplasia associated with skin lesions and endocrine disturbances [9]. Approximately 20–30% of fibrous dysplasia are polyostotic. It more frequently involves the femur, tibia, pelvis, ribs, skull, facial bones, upper extremities, lumbar spine, clavicle, and cervical spine, in decreasing order. The disease usually manifests early in life with an evident deformity of long bones, often unilateral in distribution. It has an insidious onset. Recurrent bone pain is the most common presenting skeletal symptom.

Because of the severe bone changes, spontaneous fractures are a common complication of the disease. The structural integrity of the bone is weakened and the weight-bearing areas become bowed. The curvature of the femoral neck and proximal shaft of the femur markedly increase causing a "*shepherd crook deformity*," which is a characteristic sign of the disease. Overgrowth of adjacent soft tissues may be present.

Polyostotic forms can be subclassified as follows:

1. **Jaffe-Lichtenstein** is characterized by multiple bone lesions and the skin pigmentation (café au lait) of thin light brown color. It is a mild and nonprogressive form. This type occurs in about 50% of the cases. Leg length discrepancy is very common as a result of involvement of the upper portion of the femur (hockey stick deformity). Café-au-lait pigmentation consists of well-defined, generally unilateral tan macules frequently overlying the affected bone, but predilection for the back of the neck, trunk, buttocks, thighs, and even mucosal macules also may be present. The margins of the café-au-lait spots are typically very irregular, resembling a map of the coastline of Maine.

2. **Albright's syndrome** is a polyostotic form accompanied by extensive circumscribed, predominantly ipsilateral skin pigmentations and endocrine dysfunction. The irregular pigmented melanotic spots are described as cafe-au-lait spots because of their light brown color. In addition, the female patients may exhibit precocious puberty, sometimes beginning at the age of 2 or 3 years or even younger. Vaginal bleeding is a common manifestation. Breast development and pubic hair may be apparent within the first few years of life in affected girls. The other endocrine disorders are acromegaly, hyperthyroidism, hyperparathyroidism, and hyperprolactinemia. Endocrine disturbances include those related to pituitary, thyroid, parathyroid, and ovary. In boys the disease is characterized by the early appearance of secondary sexual characteristics, i.e., gynecomastia, and occasionally by spermatogenesis. Precocious puberty may be accompanied by accelerated skeletal growth.

3. A **craniofacial form** confined to bones of the craniofacial complex. It occurs more commonly in the maxilla than mandible. Maxillary lesions may extend to involve the maxillary sinus, the zygoma, sphenoid bone, and the floor of the orbit. In case of mandibular involvement, the body of the mandible is affected mostly. It also occurs in an isolated craniofacial form where no extracranial lesion is present. It commonly affects frontal, sphenoid, maxillary, and ethmoid bone. Hypertelorism, cranial asymmetry, facial deformity, visual impairment, exophthalmos, and blindness may occur because of orbital and periorbital bone involvement. Vestibular dysfunction, tinnitus, and hearing loss may occur, if sphenoid wing and temporal bones are involved. When the cribriform plate is involved, hyposmia or anosmia may result.

13.8 Radiographic Features

Radiolucent lesions may be in the diaphysis or metaphysis with endosteal scalloping and with or without bone expansion and the absence of periosteal reaction. The lucent lesion has a thick sclerotic border and is called the **rind sign**. Frontal bone is involved more frequently than sphenoid, with obliteration of the sphenoid and frontal sinuses. Maxillary and mandibular involvement has a mixed radiolucent and radiopaque pattern, with displacement of teeth and distortion of the nasal cavities (Fig. 13.4).

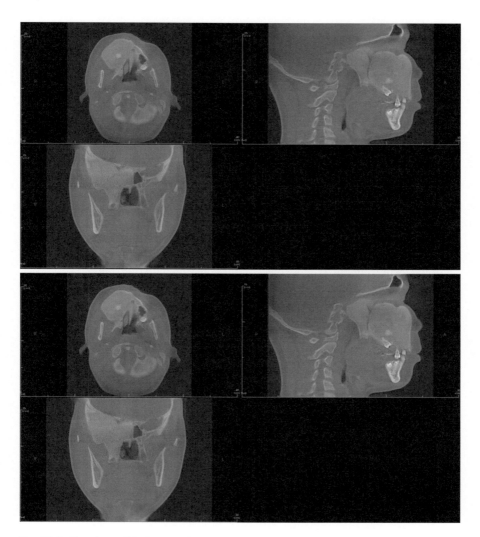

Fig. 13.4 Cone beam CT of a case of polyostotic fibrous dysplasia: The lesions are seen involving multiple bones, in this case, right side of the sphenoid, and right maxilla. (Courtesy C. Matesi, DDS)

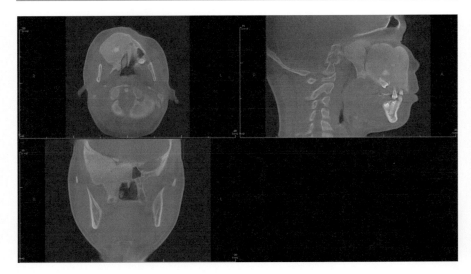

Fig. 13.4 (continued)

13.9 Differential Diagnosis

1. **Ossifying fibroma**: This lesion shows more tumor-like bone expansion (concentric growth), whereas fibrous dysplasia expands along the long axis of the bone maintaining the original outer contour. This lesion also has a distinguishing feature of thin well-defined radiolucent periphery (radiolucent rim). Displacement of the teeth from one specific epicenter is common with this lesion.
2. **Paget's disease of bone**: Occurs in older age group, involving the entire jaw and crossing the midline. Paget's disease does not encroach the antral air space. The cotton-wool appearance on the lateral cephalometric view is distinctive of Paget's disease.
3. **Osteomyelitis**: Infection, periosteal bone reaction, and bony sequestration are distinguishable features of this lesion.

13.10 Histological Features

Histological features are similar to that of monostotic FD. The lesion is composed of fibrillar connective tissue within which numerous trabeculae, in woven immature bone, irregular in shape, can be seen.

The osteocytes are quite large and collagen fibers of these trabeculae can often be observed extending into fibrous tissue. Bone formation by stellate osteoblasts can be seen, but rows of cuboidal osteoblasts lined up on the surface of the trabeculae (osteoblastic rimming) are absent. These trabeculae typically have wide osteoid seams. Osteoclastic activity may also be seen where the calcification of osteoid extends to the surface of the trabecule.

13.11 Oral Manifestations

The oral manifestations of PFD are related to severe disturbance of bony tissue. One third of the polyostotic patients have lesions in the mandible. According to Harris et al. and Church, even maxillary involvement is not rare. There may be expansion and deformity of the jaws. The eruption pattern of the teeth is disturbed because of loss of support of the developing teeth. The endocrine disturbance also may alter the time of eruption of the teeth.

13.12 Treatment

Mild cases may be treated surgically. Severe forms are treated with X-ray radiation with some success, but it is hazardous because of the possibility of development of induced osteosarcomas.

References

1. Lichtenstein L. Polyostotic fibrous dysplasia. Arch Surg. 1938;36:874–98.
2. Albright F, Butler AM, Hampton AO, Smith P. Syndrome characterized by osteitis fibrosa disseminata, etc. N Engl J Med. 1937;216:727.
3. Uehlinger E. Osteofibrosis deformans juvenalis. Virchows Archiv. 1940;306:255.
4. Lichtenstein L, Jaffe HL. Fibrous dysplasia of bone. Arch Pathol. 1942;33:777.
5. Falconer MA, Cope CL. Fibrous dysplasia of bone. Q J Med. 1942;11:121.
6. Windholz F. Cranial manifestations of fibrous dysplasia of bone. Am J Roentgenol. 1947;58:51.
7. Pierce AM, Wilson DF, Enneking WF. Inherited craniofacial fibrous dysplasia. Oral Surg Oral Med Oral Pathol. 1985;60:403–9.
8. Zohar Y, Grausbord R, Shabtai F, Talmi Y. Fibrous dysplasia and cherubism as a hereditary disease. Follow up of four generations. J Craniomaxillofac Surg. 1989;17:340–4.
9. Jaffe HL, Lichtenstein L. Solitary unicameral bone cyst with emphasis on the Roentgen picture, the pathologic appearance, and the pathogenesis. Arch Surg. 1942;44:1004–25.

Cherubism

14

(Familial Fibrous Dysplasia of the Jaws, Disseminated Juvenile Fibrous Dysplasia, Familial Multilocular Cystic Disease of the Jaws, Familial Fibrous Swelling of the Jaws)

Contents

14.1	Clinical Features	54
14.2	Grading System	54
14.3	Oral Manifestations	55
14.4	Radiographic Features	55
14.5	Differential Diagnosis	56
14.6	Histological Features	56
14.7	Treatment	57
References		58

Cherubism is an uncommon, benign fibro-osseous lesion which causes a progressive, painless, symmetrical expansion of the jaws. It is primarily found in the mandible. The disease was first described in 1933 by Jones [1], who called it familial multilocular disease of the jaws. He coined the term cherubism, because the affected persons resembled the figure in Renaissance art that had a round full-face appearance and upturned eyes. Peter reported a family with no less than 20 affected members. Zohar et al. were able to trace, in an unbroken line through four generations, family members who showed either fibrous dysplasia or cherubism. According to the WHO classification, cherubism belongs to a group of nonneoplastic bone lesions affecting only the jaws. It is a rare, benign condition with autosomal dominant inheritance, and it is one of the very few genetically determined osteoclastic lesions in the human body. It appears to have 100% penetrance in males and only 50–70% penetrance in females with 2:1 male predominance.

There is great variation in the clinical expression. Although the condition is known to be hereditary, in some cases there has been no detectable family history. Although it usually occurs bilaterally, there have also been cases of unilateral involvement, perhaps because of incomplete penetration or new mutations. Some investigators believe that cherubism arises from the mutation of a non-sex-linked

© The Author(s), under exclusive license to Springer Nature Singapore Pte Ltd. 2024
K. Paiwal et al., *Handbook of Oral and Maxillofacial Giant Cell Lesions*,
https://doi.org/10.1007/978-981-97-2863-3_14

gene responsible for the development of the jaw bones. The specific gene related to cherubism was located on chromosome 4p 16.3, which encodes the SH3-binding protein, SH3 BP2. This protein controls the signal transduction pathway which in turn regulates normal osteoblastic and osteoclastic activity in tooth-bearing area of the jaw.

14.1 Clinical Features

Affected children are normal at birth and are without clinically or radiographically evident disease until 14 months to 3 years of age. At that time, symmetric enlargement of the jaw begins. Typically, the earlier the lesion appears, the more rapidly it progresses. The self-limited bone growth usually begins to slow down when the patient reaches 5 years of age and stops by the age of 12–15 years. At puberty the lesions begin to regress. Jaw remodeling continues through the third decade of life, at the end of which the clinical abnormality may be subtle. The signs and symptoms depend on the severity of the condition and range from clinically or radiologically undetectable features, i.e., mandibular and maxillary overgrowth with respiratory obstruction, to vision as well as hearing impairment and difficulty in speech and swallowing.

14.2 Grading System

Arnott [2] suggested the following grading system for the lesions of cherubism: Grade I is characterized by involvement of both mandibular ascending rami, Grade II by involvement of both maxillary tuberosities as well as the mandibular ascending rami, and Grade III by McCune-Albright syndrome involvement of the whole maxilla and mandible except the coronoid process and condyles.

The jaw lesions are usually painless and symmetric and have florid maxillary involvement. The lesions are firm on palpation, non-tender, and bilaterally symmetrical. The most commonly involved are the molar to coronoid regions, the condyles always being spared and often associated with cervical lymphadenopathy. Enlargement of the cervical lymph nodes contributes to the patient's full-face appearance and is said to be caused by lymphoid hyperplasia with fibrosis. The lymph nodes become enlarged before the patient reaches 6 years of age, decrease in size after the age of 8 years, and are rarely enlarged after the age of 12 years. Intraoral swelling of the alveolar ridges may occur. When the maxillary ridge is involved, the palate assumes a V shape. A rim of sclera may be visible beneath the iris, giving the classic "eye to heaven" appearance.

14.3 Oral Manifestations

Numerous dental abnormalities, such as agenesis of the second and third molars of the mandible, displacement of the teeth, premature exfoliation of the primary teeth, delayed eruption of the permanent teeth, and transpositions as well as rotation of the teeth, have been reported. In severe cases, tooth resorption may also occur. The deciduous dentition may be shed prematurely, beginning as early as 3 years of age. The permanent dentition is often defective, with absence of numerous teeth, displacement, and lack of eruption of those present. The oral mucosa is usually intact and of normal color. Although cherubism was initially described as a familial disease affecting the jaws, cases without any apparent hereditary origin have been reported. In a few cases, cherubism has been described as being connected with other diseases and conditions such as **Noonan's syndrome**, a lesion in the humerus, gingival fibromatosis, psychomotor retardation, orbital involvement, and obstructive sleep apnea. The association between these two rare inherited diseases suggests that these are independent diseases that may be transmitted by genes closely linked on the same chromosome.

14.4 Radiographic Features

Radiographically, cherubism is characterized by bilateral multilocular, radiolucent, cystic expansion of the jaws. Early lesions occur in the posterior body of the mandible and the ascending rami. Maxillary lesions may occur at the same time but escape early radiographic detection because of overlap of the sinus and nasal cavities. The periphery of the lesions is well-defined and corticated. The internal septa appear wispy and fine similar to central giant cell granuloma. Displacement of the inferior alveolar canal has been reported. The teeth are displaced anteriorly toward the midline. The developing teeth may be malformed and fail to erupt giving the radiographic appearance referred to as *floating tooth syndrome* (Fig. 14.1a, b). With adulthood, the cystic areas in the jaws regress and are replaced by irregular patchy sclerosis.

There may be classic, but nonspecific, ground glass appearance because of the small, tightly compressed trabecular pattern similar to fibrous dysplasia.

Fig. 14.1 (a) A reconstructed panoramic view showing bilateral multilocular, hypodense, cystic lesion of the jaws. Note anterior displacement of the unerupted lower second molars (Courtesy AZ. Syed, BDS, MHA, MS, Dipl. ABOMR). (b) Coronal view of the same patient showing bilateral multilocular, hypodense, expansile lesions of the jaws

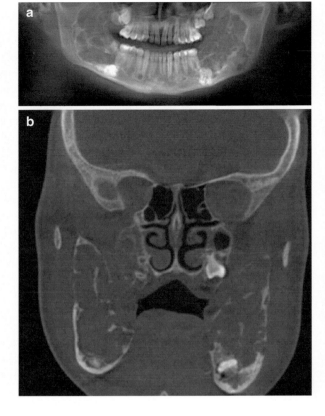

14.5 Differential Diagnosis

1. **Nevoid basal cell carcinoma**: Multiple jaw lesions (odontogenic keratocysts) with minimal expansion are seen. This syndrome shows systemic manifestations such as ocular hypertelorism, bifid rib, falx cerebri calcification, and palmar and plantar pits.
2. **Fibrous dysplasia**: Mostly unilateral presentation and rarely crosses the midline. Changes the bone pattern without teeth displacement.
3. **Central giant cell granuloma**: Mostly single lesion and located anteriorly in the jaws. This lesion doesn't regress in adulthood.

14.6 Histological Features

Histologic examination of the lesions usually reveals numerous multinucleated giant cells. These multinucleated cells show strong positivity for tartrate-resistant acid phosphatase, which is characteristic of osteoclasts. The collagenous stroma,

Fig. 14.2 Image 4×

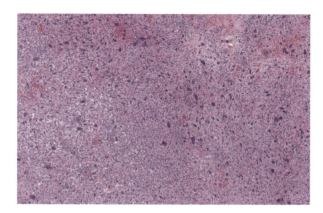

Fig. 14.3 Image 10×

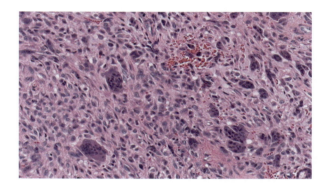

which contains a large number of spindle-shaped fibroblasts, is considered unique because of its water-logged, granular nature (Figs. 14.2 and 14.3). Numerous small vessels are present. The capillaries exhibit large endothelial cells and perivascular cuffing. The eosinophilic cuffing appears to be specific to cherubism. However, these deposits are not present in many cases and their absence does not exclude the diagnosis of cherubism. Older, resolving lesions of cherubism show an increase in fibrous tissue, a decrease in the number of giant cells, and formation of new bone. The microscopic findings seldom permit a specific diagnosis of cherubism in the absence of clinical and radiological information.

14.7 Treatment

As Laskin stated, "the treatment should be based on the known natural course of the disease and the clinical behavior of the individual case." Surgery to correct the jaw deformities of cherubism is rarely indicated. If necessary, surgery is usually undertaken after puberty, when the remission phase of the lesions has been reached, unless aesthetic considerations or severe functional problems justify earlier treatment. Although exacerbation has sometimes been reported after surgery, it is believed that surgery ultimately accelerates the involution process.

References

1. Jones WA. Familial multilocular cystic disease of the jaws. Am J Cancer. 1933;17:946–50.
2. Arnott DG. Cherubism—an initial unilateral presentation. Br J Oral Surg. 1978;16:38–46.

Paget's Disease

15

(Paget's Disease of Bone, Osteitis Deformans)

Contents

15.1	Clinical Features	59
15.2	Oral Manifestations	60
15.3	Radiographic Features	61
15.4	Differential Diagnosis	62
15.5	Laboratory Findings	62
15.6	Histological Features	62
15.7	Treatment and Prognosis	63

Paget's disease is a metabolic disorder affecting the bones. It causes a malfunction in the normal process of bone remodeling. Paget's disease is named after Sir James Paget, an English surgeon who described the clinical course of this disorder and originally named the condition "*osteitis deformans*," as he believed the disease was caused by chronic inflammation.

Paget's disease of bone is characterized by enhanced resorption of bone by giant multinucleated osteoclasts with formation of disorganized woven bone by osteoblasts. This process evolves through various phases of activity, followed by a quiescent stage. Hence, Paget's disease typically consists of the following three phases: (1) lytic, (2) mixed lytic and blastic, and (3) sclerotic or burned out.

15.1 Clinical Features

The prevalence of Paget's disease increases with age. Paget's disease is recognized most commonly after the age of 50 years and is rarely diagnosed in people younger than 40 years. By the ninth decade of life, prevalence reaches nearly 10% of the peer group. The male to female ratio is approximately 1:1.

© The Author(s), under exclusive license to Springer Nature Singapore Pte Ltd. 2024
K. Paiwal et al., *Handbook of Oral and Maxillofacial Giant Cell Lesions*,
https://doi.org/10.1007/978-981-97-2863-3_15

A large number of patients in the community are asymptomatic or have mild/unrecognized symptoms. Paget's disease has a predilection for the axial skeleton and may be widespread at the time of diagnosis. The condition commonly affects the pelvis and spine, particularly the lumbar spine with a frequency of 30–75%.

Pain is the most common presenting symptom. It may arise from bone affected by pagetic lesions, arthritic or distorted joint architecture, fissure or complete fracture, and neurological compression syndromes. The bone pain is perceived as a dull constant aching pain deep below the soft tissues. It may persist or exacerbate during the night. The involved bones become warm to touch because of the increased vascularity.

Other typical findings may include the following: pathologic fractures commonly result from weakened pagetic bone; nonspecific headaches, impaired hearing, and tinnitus are common symptoms with skull involvement. The patient's hat size may increase or change due to skeletal deformity and enlargement, especially of the skull bones. Cranial nerve palsies can affect nerves other than the auditory nerve. Change in vision can occur secondary to optic nerve involvement. Back and neck pain are common complaints, as Paget's disease frequently affects the spine, especially the lumbar and sacral regions. Softened bone at the base of the skull may lead to platybasia, the descent of the cranium onto the cervical spine. Progressive pain, paresthesia, limb paresis, gait difficulties (waddling gait), or bowel and bladder incontinence may be caused by compression of the spinal cord or spinal nerve secondary to platybasia or vertebral fractures. Nausea, dizziness, syncope, ataxia, incontinence, and dementia can be observed with hydrocephalus, basilar invagination, and cerebellar or brain stem compression syndromes.

Involvement of the facial bones is occasionally seen. It has sometimes been called *leontiasis ossea* (lion-like facies), but because this term is nonspecific, Drury advocated discontinuing its use in referring to this disease.

15.2 Oral Manifestations

Involvement of the jaws in osteitis deformans is a rather common occurrence. There is predilection for the maxilla; the ratio of involvement of the maxilla to mandible is approximately 2.3:1. The maxilla exhibits progressive enlargement; the alveolar ridge becomes widened and the palate is flattened. The teeth become loose and migrate, producing spacing in between the teeth. When the mandible is involved, the findings are similar but usually not as severe as in the maxilla. As the disease progresses, the mouth may remain open, exposing the teeth because the lips are too small to cover the enlarged jaw.

Edentulous patients with dentures commonly complain of an inability to wear their appliances because of increasing tightness due to expansion of the jaw. The dentures may be remade periodically. When the jaws are involved by Paget's disease, there may be involvement of the skull also.

15.3 Radiographic Features

Paget's disease has sometimes been described as a disorder characterized by an initial phase of demineralization and softening followed by a bizarre, dysplastic type of re-ossification not related to functional requirements, the two processes taking place simultaneously or alternatively. These destructive lesions may be multiple and diffuse or isolated. The isolated lesion in the skull, when large, is sometimes referred to as "osteoporosis circumscripta." The osteoblastic areas, which appear as opacities, tend to be patchy in distribution. This patchiness has been termed a "cotton-wool" appearance and is especially well demonstrated in the skull and jaws (Fig. 15.1a, b). In the skull, the diploic spaces may be enlarged with areas of demineralization and sclerosis. The cortical bone may be abnormally thickened as well. Skull enlargement may resemble a Scottish hat, termed as "Tam o' Shanter" skull. Platybasia, frontal bossing, and basilar invagination may be present.

Although the disease is usually bilateral, it may show evidence of only unilateral involvement of the jaw, especially early in the course of the disease. The entire jaw will be involved with or without enlargement. The teeth show a rather pronounced hypercementosis and loss of a well-defined lamina dura. Root resorption has been reported in some cases, but this is unusual.

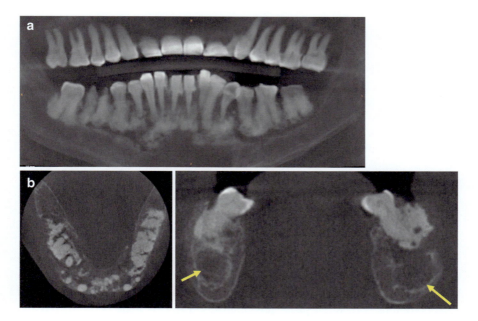

Fig. 15.1 (**a**) CBCT reconstructed panoramic view of a patient with Paget's disease showing cotton-wool bone pattern in the entire mandible. (**b**) CBCT axial and coronal sections of the same patient showing mixed low- and high-density areas throughout the entire mandibular body. Well-defined areas of low density are seen bilaterally representing simple bone cavities within the lesion (yellow arrows). (Courtesy of Sadaksharam J, MDS, PhD, Nagarajan N, MDS)

15.4 Differential Diagnosis

1. **Fibrous dysplasia**: Occurs in younger age groups with unilateral presentation. Rarely crosses the midline. Fibrous dysplasia can involve the air space, whereas Paget's disease does not.
2. **Florid osseous dysplasia**: Lesions are located above the inferior alveolar canal and most commonly have a radiolucent capsule.
3. **Metabolic bone diseases**: Both lesions are bilateral. However, no expansion is noted with metabolic disease.

15.5 Laboratory Findings

The serum calcium and serum phosphorus levels are usually within normal limits even in cases of advanced osteitis deformans. The serum alkaline phosphatase level may be elevated to over 250 Bodansky units. The serum acid phosphatase level is not increased. Urinary hydroxyproline levels are elevated as they reflect increased osteoclastic activity and bone resorption.

15.6 Histological Features

The initial osteolytic phase is marked by disordered areas of resorption by an increased number of large osteoclasts. These abnormal osteoclasts may contain up to 100 nuclei. The subsequent osteoblastic phase follows with haphazard laying of new bone matrix and formation of woven bone without patterns of stress in between. Repeated episodes of bone removal and formation result in the appearance of many small irregularly shaped bone fragments that appear to be joined in a jigsaw or mosaic pattern with deeply staining hematoxyphilic reversal lines. This pattern is the histologic hallmark of Paget's disease. As the disease progresses, the osteoblastic phase predominates and excessive abnormal bone formation occurs, causing more compact and dense bone. The pagetic bone is coarse and fibrous, with avidity for calcium and phosphorus. Marrow spaces are filled with loose and highly vascularized connective tissue. The hypervascular bone combined with cutaneous vasodilation causes an increase in the regional blood flow and accounts for the rise in skin temperature.

The normal trabecular appearance is distorted with a mosaic pattern of irregular cement lines joining areas of lamellar bone. Pagetic bone shows no tendency to form Haversian systems. Eventually, the osteoblastic activity diminishes and an osteoporotic or burned-out phase predominates. The new bone is disordered and poorly mineralized and lacks structural integrity. The proliferation of bone and concomitant hypercementosis sometimes result in obliteration of the periodontal ligament space.

15.7 Treatment and Prognosis

Calcitonin can be used which suppresses bone resorption. Bisphosphonates have also been used with some success. Prognosis of the patients with Paget's disease is good if the treatment is administered before major changes in the bones have occurred.

Giant Cell Tumor of Bone

16

Contents

16.1 Pathogenesis.. 65
16.2 Clinical Features.. 66

Giant cell tumor (GCT) of bone is also known as *osteoclastoma*. They are fairly common tumors, accounting for about 20% of all benign tumors of the bone. Most cases arise in the epiphyses of long bones, particularly the distal femur, proximal tibia, proximal humerus, and distal radius. Giant cell tumors are true neoplasms that exhibit a wide spectrum of biologic behavior from benign to malignant. The relationship between this lesion and central giant cell granuloma is controversial. Most regard the giant cell tumor as a distinct entity from central giant cell granuloma, acknowledging the very rare occurrence of giant cell tumors within the jaws.

Giant cell tumor is a primary benign tumor but may evolve into a malignant tumor, usually after irradiation.

16.1 Pathogenesis

Giant cell tumor of bone is a distinctive neoplasm of undifferentiated cells. Multinucleated giant cells apparently result from fusion of the proliferating mononuclear cells, and although they are a constant and prominent part of this tumor, the giant cells are probably of less significance than the mononuclear cells. The exact cell of origin of this neoplasm is still unknown. Several immunohistochemical studies have suggested that the mononuclear cells are of histiocytic origin and that the giant cells arise from their fusion.

© The Author(s), under exclusive license to Springer Nature Singapore Pte
Ltd. 2024
K. Paiwal et al., *Handbook of Oral and Maxillofacial Giant Cell Lesions*,
https://doi.org/10.1007/978-981-97-2863-3_16

16.2 Clinical Features

They occur most often between the ages of 20 and 40 years, with a slight female predominance. Giant cell tumors, although rare, have been reported in the jaws. Other sites of involvement in the head and neck include the sphenoid, ethmoid, and temporal bones. Giant cell tumors are most often seen in the third and fourth decades of life with peak incidence in third decade.

This lesion may exhibit a wide range of biologic behavior and thus may present a variety of clinical features. Benign variants may exhibit slow growth and bone expansion. Rapid malignant variety or large tumors may produce rapid growth. Pain of variable severity is almost always a predominant symptom. Less common symptoms are weakness, limitation of motion of the joint, and pathological fracture.

Malignant Giant Cell Tumor

17

Contents

17.1 Radiographic Features.. 67
17.2 Histological Features... 67
17.3 Treatment and Prognosis.. 69

Giant cell tumors are known to evolve into malignant tumors. McGrath (1972) classified such tumors into three types: primary, evolutionary, and secondary. "Primary" is for tumors that are malignant from outset, "evolutionary" for typical tumors that progress to a malignant form within a short period, and "secondary" for typical tumors that undergo sarcomatous changes after a relatively long symptom-free period and usually develop after irradiation (postirradiation malignancy).

17.1 Radiographic Features

The radiographic presentation of benign lesions varies from small unilocular radiolucencies to large multilocular entities with well- or ill-defined margins. Cortical perforation and root resorption may be observed. When the lesion presents with areas of bone destruction showing aggressiveness, malignant transformation should be suspected.

17.2 Histological Features

On gross inspection the lesion is well circumscribed and often has a granular hemorrhagic appearance. The expanded portion is partially or completely encased in a thin shell of bone. The neoplastic tissue is firm and friable. It is often grayish, with

© The Author(s), under exclusive license to Springer Nature Singapore Pte
Ltd. 2024
K. Paiwal et al., *Handbook of Oral and Maxillofacial Giant Cell Lesions*,
https://doi.org/10.1007/978-981-97-2863-3_17

either a pinkish or a brownish tint. Focal areas of cystic degeneration of yellow-brown color and hemorrhagic areas that are red or dark brown, depending on the age of the hemorrhage, are usually present.

The microscopic hallmark of this neoplasm is the presence of a large number of multinucleated giant cells that are regularly scattered throughout the tumor mass (Fig. 17.1). The giant cells of this neoplasm have an abundant acidophilic cytoplasm and as many as 100 nuclei. Their light microscopic, enzymatic, histochemical, and fine structural features are similar to those of normal osteoclasts. Thus, acid phosphatase activity is very high and a large number of mitochondria are present in the cytoplasm. Because of these similarities, giant cell tumor of bone is also known as osteoclastoma.

The second microscopic component of the giant cell tumor is the stromal *cell*. Although far less spectacular than the giant cell when examined under the microscope, it is probably the basic tumor element. It is certainly more important numerically than the giant cell. The relative number and appearance of these stromal cells correlate with the clinical evolution. In locally aggressive and metastasizing lesions, one often gets the impression that the stromal cell component has taken over the neoplasm.

The stromal cells of a typical giant cell tumor are medium-sized and oval or spindle-shaped, with rather plump nuclei and ill-defined acidophilic cytoplasm (Fig. 17.2). Mononuclear macrophages are also present in large numbers, but they probably are nonneoplastic and an expression of the host reaction to the tumor. The stroma is richly vascularized and contains a small amount of collagen. In about a third of the cases, foci of osteoid or bone formation of reactive appearance are found. Under the electron microscope, the stromal cells are seen to contain a well-developed granular endoplasmic reticulum. Their appearance is reminiscent of a fibroblast or an osteoblast.

Fig. 17.1 Image 4×

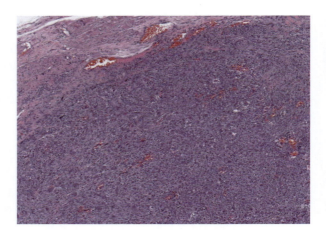

Fig. 17.2 Image 10×

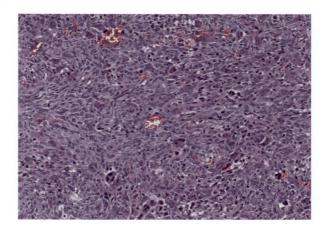

17.3 Treatment and Prognosis

Surgical excision is the treatment of choice for giant cell tumors. Giant cell tumors are aggressive lesions. As much as 60% recur after curettage and about 10% result in distant metastasis, usually to the lungs.

Hodgkin's Disease

18

Hodgkin's Lymphoma, Malignant Lymphoma

Contents

18.1	Clinical Features	71
18.2	Oral Manifestations	72
18.3	Histological Features	72
18.4	Radiographic Features	73
18.5	Differential Diagnosis	74
18.6	Treatment and Prognosis	74

Thomas Hodgkin first described Hodgkin's disease in 1832. It is a potentially curable malignant lymphoma with distinct histology, biologic behavior, and clinical characteristics.

The etiology of HD is unknown. Infectious agents, especially the Epstein-Barr virus (EBV), may be involved in the pathogenesis. Patients with HIV infection have a higher incidence of HD compared to the population without HIV infection. Genetic predisposition may play a role in the pathogenesis.

18.1 Clinical Features

Age-specific incidence rates have a bimodal distribution in both genders, peaking in young adults (aged 15–34 years) and older individuals (>55 years). HD is more common in males than in females, particularly evident in children.

The first manifestation in the majority of cases is painless enlargement of one or more cervical lymph nodes. Palpable painless lymphadenopathy occurs in the cervical area (60–80%), the axilla (6–20%), the inguinal area (6–20%), and Waldeyer ring or occipital nodes. The nodes are usually firm and rubbery in consistency and the overlying skin is normal.

© The Author(s), under exclusive license to Springer Nature Singapore Pte Ltd. 2024
K. Paiwal et al., *Handbook of Oral and Maxillofacial Giant Cell Lesions*,
https://doi.org/10.1007/978-981-97-2863-3_18

Constitutional symptoms such as unexplained weight loss, fever, and night sweats are present in about 40% of patients. Chest pain, cough, and/or shortness of breath may be present due to a large mediastinal mass or lung involvement. Rarely, hemoptysis is observed. Alcohol-induced pain at sites of nodal disease is specific for HD. Patient may present with pruritus or intermittent fever. Back, abdominal, or bone pain occurs rarely.

18.2 Oral Manifestations

Hodgkin's disease is primarily a disease of lymph nodes and the oral cavity could be involved secondarily. A case of Hodgkin's disease secondarily involving the mandible and overlying alveolar mucosa has been reported by Forman and Wesson.

18.3 Histological Features

1. **Nodular sclerosis Hodgkin's disease** comprises 60–80% of all cases. The morphology shows a nodular pattern. The broad bands of fibrosis divide the node into "nodules." The capsule is thickened. The characteristic cell is the lacunar-type RS cell, which has a monolobated or multilobulated nucleus and a small nucleolus with abundant and pale cytoplasm. NS frequently is observed in adolescents and young adults and usually involves the mediastinum and other supra-diaphragmatic sites.
2. **Mixed-cellularity Hodgkin's disease** comprises 15–30%. Histologically, the infiltrate is usually diffuse. RS cells are of the classic type (large, with bilobate, double, or multiple nuclei and a large eosinophilic inclusion like nucleolus). It commonly affects the abdominal lymph nodes and spleen.
3. **Lymphocyte-depleted Hodgkin's disease** makes up less than 1%. The infiltrate in lymphocyte-depleted Hodgkin's disease (LDHD) is diffuse and often appears hypocellular. Large numbers of RS cells and bizarre sarcomatous variants are present. It is associated with older age and HIV positivity. Patients usually present with advanced-stage disease.

4. **Lymphocyte-rich classic Hodgkin's disease** comprises 5%. In this type of HD, RS cells of the classic or lacunar type are observed, with a background infiltrate of lymphocytes. Clinically, the presentation and survival patterns are similar to those for mixed-cellularity Hodgkin's disease.
5. **Nodular lymphocyte-predominant Hodgkin's disease** constitutes 5%. A variant of RS cells, the lymphocytic and histiocytic (L&H) cells, or popcorn cells (their nuclei resemble an exploded kernel of corn) are seen within a background of inflammatory cells, predominantly benign lymphocytes.

18.4 Radiographic Features

The radiographic presentation of the lesions is not specific. It shows an ill-defined, infiltrative, radiolucent area with minimal expansion (Fig. 18.1). Cortical perforation and root resorption may be observed. When the lesion presents with areas of bone destruction with minimal expansion, malignant symptoms should be suspected.

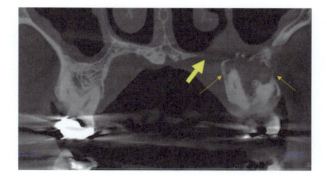

Fig. 18.1 A cropped coronal view for patients with NHL. Please note the bony destruction in the left hard palate (yellow arrow) and the minimal expansion (orange arrows). (Courtesy A.Z. Syed, BDS, MHA, MS, Dipl. ABOMR)

18.5 Differential Diagnosis

1. **Squamous cell carcinomas**: Similar radiographically. Clinical finding of soft tissue lesions favors squamous cell carcinoma.
2. **Multiple myeloma**: Occurs in older age groups, multiple well-defined non-corticated lesions.
3. **Metastatic carcinoma**: Occurs in older age groups. Clinical history of primary lesions can help to differentiate this lesion.

18.6 Treatment and Prognosis

Radiation therapy and combination chemotherapy have been clearly shown to be effective in the management of Hodgkin's disease. The most important prognostic determinants are the histologic type and the clinical stage of the disease. The lymphocyte predominant type has the most favorable prognosis, followed by nodular sclerosis, mixed cellularity, and lymphocyte depletion, the least favorable. Localized (Stage I) disease has a much better prognosis than disseminated (Stage IV) disease.

Aneurysmal Bone Cyst

19

Contents

19.1   Pathogenesis.. 76
19.2   Clinical Features.. 77
19.3   Radiological Features... 78
19.4   Differential Diagnosis.. 80
19.5   Histological Features... 80
19.6   Treatment.. 82
References... 82

The aneurysmal bone cyst (ABC) is an uncommon lesion which has been found in most bones of the skeleton. Jaffe and Lichtenstein were the first to recognize ABC as an intraosseous, osteolytic lesion chiefly affecting the metaphyseal region of long bones and vertebrae. The term "aneurysmal bone cyst" was suggested by Jaffe and Lichtenstein [1], the word "aneurysmal" to emphasize the "blown-out," distended contour of the affected bone and the words "bone cyst" to underscore that when the lesion is entered through a thin shell of bone, it appears largely as a blood-filled cavity.

According to Clough and Price [2], the majority of lesions occur in long bones and in the spine. Bernier and Bhaskar [3] described the first case of ABC involving the craniofacial skeleton. Only 1.9% of all ABCs occur in the jaws, representing 1.5% of all nonodontogenic cysts.

The **World Health Organization** defines aneurysmal bone cyst (ABC) as "a benign tumor-like lesion with an expanding osteolytic lesion consisting of blood-filled spaces of variable size separated by connective tissue septa containing trabeculae of osteoid tissue and osteoclast giant cells." Although benign, ABC can be a rapidly growing and destructive bone lesion. The expansile nature of this lesion can cause pain, swelling, deformity, perforation or disruption of cortical plates, neurological symptoms (depending on its location), and pathologic fracture.

© The Author(s), under exclusive license to Springer Nature Singapore Pte Ltd. 2024
K. Paiwal et al., *Handbook of Oral and Maxillofacial Giant Cell Lesions*, https://doi.org/10.1007/978-981-97-2863-3_19

19.1 Pathogenesis

The pathogenesis of the aneurysmal bone cyst is controversial and a number of theories have been proposed. The original cases reported by Jaffe and Lichtenstein [1] were in the long bones and showed eccentric bone expansion indicating a juxta-cortical or subperiosteal lesion.

Subsequently, it has become apparent that the aneurysmal bone cyst may have a juxtacortical or intramedullary location. Kransdorf and Sweet [4] have led to the concept of aneurysmal bone cyst being the end result of a common pathophysiologi-cal process with a variety of causes. Juxtacortical lesions that are found in a subperi-osteal location are thought to be primarily of traumatic origin, whereas intramedullary lesions reflect secondary change within pre-existing lesions. Juxtacortical lesions have not been reported in the head and neck, and although trauma has been postu-lated, there is little evidence to support this as a cause of jaw lesions. Kransdorf and Sweet [4] suggested that the cysts may result from a vascular disturbance in the form of sudden venous occlusion or the development of an arteriovenous shunt. This would usually occur in more vascular, newly formed parts of the immature skeleton and in a pre-existing lesion.

The concept of aneurysmal bone cyst as a secondary phenomenon occurring in a pre-existing lesion has been validated by multiple investigators; in approximately one third (29–35%) of cases, the pre-existing lesion can be identified. The most common of these is giant cell tumor, which accounts for 19–39% of those cases in which the preceding lesion is found. Other common precursor lesions include osteo-blastoma, angioma, and chondroblastoma. Less common lesions include fibrous dysplasia, fibroxanthoma (nonossifying fibroma), chondromyxoid fibroma, solitary bone cyst, fibrous histiocytoma, eosinophilic granuloma, radiation osteitis, osteo-sarcoma, trauma (including fracture), fibrosarcoma, and even metastatic carcinoma.

Other investigators have proposed two forms of aneurysmal bone cyst, those in which the lesion is secondary to an identifiable precursor and a "primary aneurys-mal bone cyst" in which no pre-existing lesion is identified.

Struthers and Shear [5] suggested that the initiating change in the primary lesion appeared to be the microcyst. They pointed out that the formation of microcysts in fibrous dysplasia had been described by Geschickter and Copeland [6], Jaffe [7], and Fisher [8]. The central giant cell granuloma has a propensity to form microcysts because of its loose, edematous, fibrillar connective tissue stroma in which lie many thin-walled blood vessels and extravasated erythrocytes. Microcyst formation is facilitated by localized areas of necrosis in the stroma brought about by stagnation and ischemia. The resulting microcysts are lined by stromal connective tissue and in giant cell lesions, multinucleated giant cells may form part of their margins. They enlarge by further stromal breakdown and coalesce with each other. Loss of stromal support leads to dilatation and rupture of the thin-walled vessels which leads to hemorrhage into the stroma followed by the microcyst formation. An association of dilated blood vessels and microcysts is frequently observed.

Once a vascular connection is established between a larger vessel and a microcyst, hemodynamic pressure participates in its enlargement, and little supportive resistance is offered if the surrounding stroma is loose and edematous. The spaces now assume the dimensions of macrocysts which are surrounded by a layer of compressed stroma, and these multiple expanding blood-filled cysts produce a pressure resorption of bone. Endosteal resorption of the cortical plates occurs ultimately and once these are breached, a "blowout" of the lesion, covered with periosteum, occurs. A layer of periosteal new bone may be deposited to form a thin shell covering the aneurysmal bone cyst.

Struthers and Shear [9] were of the opinion that a malignant lesion was less likely to produce the classic clinicopathological features of an aneurysmal bone cyst because of its tendency to break out of bone. Levy et al. [10] stated that the rare development of aneurysmal bone cyst in malignant lesions probably explains the so-called malignant form of the cyst occasionally reported in the literature.

To conclude this discussion of the possible pathogenesis of the aneurysmal bone cyst, it should be stated that there are a number of authorities who dispute the theory that the cyst is a secondary phenomenon.

Chromosomal translocation t(16;17)(q22;p13) can be seen as a recurring abnormality in aneurysmal bone cyst indicating that some of the lesions are neoplastic. Nonrandom rearrangements of chromosome bands 16q22 and 17p13 are observed in solid variant of ABC and extraosseous ABC suggesting that the entire spectrum of ABCs probably shares a common pathogenesis.

19.2 Clinical Features

The aneurysmal bone cyst is generally a lesion of young persons, predominantly occurring under the age of 20 years. The lesion can be encountered in adults as well. ABCs are found more frequently in the mandible than the maxilla (3:1) with preponderance for the body, ramus, and angle of the mandible. Involvement of other bones of the face such as zygoma and zygomatic arch has also been reported.

There is no significant predilection for either gender. However recent studies have indicated an increased incidence in females.

The lesions are usually tender or painful, particularly upon motion, and this soreness may limit movement of the affected bone. Swelling over the area of bone involvement is also common.

Occasionally, there is a history of recent displacement of teeth, which remain vital. When the lesion perforates the cortex and is covered by periosteum or only a thin shell of bone, it may exhibit springiness or eggshell crackling, but is not pulsatile. Bruits are not heard. Patients may complain of some degree of trismus or temporomandibular joint pain. This can be attributed to the physical impingement of the lesion on the joint capsule.

Gross findings at the time of operation are characteristic. Upon entering the lesion, excessive bleeding is encountered, the blood "welling up" from the tissue. The tissue has been described as resembling a blood-soaked sponge with large pores representing the cavernous spaces of the lesion. In manometric studies by Biesecker and his associates, some of the cysts had elevated vascular pressures as high as arteriolar levels. According to Shafer a history of traumatic injury preceding development of the lesion may often be obtained.

The cyst contains a variable amount of soft tissue consisting of friable vascular tissue which subdivides the cavity into a number of blood-filled locules. Part of the lesion may contain areas of more solid tissue. These may represent either areas of repair or remnants of a pre-existing lesion. No direct communication with any vessels can be demonstrated at operation.

19.3 Radiological Features

The lesion has a characteristic "ballooning" growth pattern with typical "blown-out" cortical expansion (Fig. 19.1). It presents with well-defined and thinned out cortical borders. Wispy, granular septa oriented at right angle to the outer cortex give it a multilocular appearance. CT with contrast will reveal multiple fluid-filled spaces. Fluid level is a typical radiographic feature which occurs due to the separation of two fluids of differing densities.

Teeth may be displaced, and root resorption may be present. Top differential diagnosis includes central giant cell granuloma which might be less expansile when compared to aneurysmal bone cyst.

19.3 Radiological Features

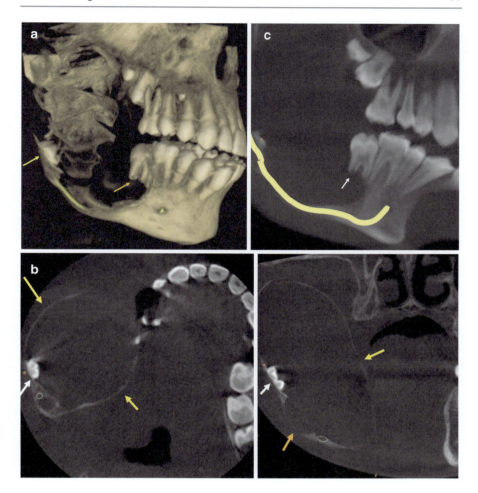

Fig. 19.1 (**a**) 3D reconstructed CBCT image of a case of aneurysmal bone cyst showing a destructive lesion occupying the right mandibular body and ramus. Note the inferior displacement of the unerupted developing third molar (yellow arrow) and the inferior alveolar canal (marked in yellow). The root of the second molar is resorbed (orange arrow) (courtesy S. Jayachandran, MDS, PhD, MAMS, MBA and N. Nagarajan, MDS). (**b**) CBCT axial and coronal images of the same patient. A well-defined, corticated, expansile, unilocular, hypodense lesion is seen occupying the entire right body and ramus of the mandible. Note the ballooning expansion and thinning of the buccal and lingual cortical plates (yellow arrow) with scalloping in some areas (orange arrows). The mandibular canal (marked in yellow) is displaced inferiorly and laterally. Note the displacement of the unerupted developing third molar (white arrow). (**c**) CBCT parasagittal section of the same patient showing root resorption of the second molar (white arrow)

19.4 Differential Diagnosis

1. **Ameloblastoma**: Occurs usually in older population, located posteriorly in the jaws, with coarse septa and more prominent cortical border.
2. **Central giant cell granuloma**: Usually located anteriorly in the jaws. Radiological and histopathological findings are similar to ABC. However, more expansion is suspected with ABC.
3. **Brown tumors of hyperparathyroidism**: Occur in patients with underlying thyroid problem (hyperparathyroidism) and older patients. Multiple lesions can be seen.
4. **Cherubism**: Occur usually in younger age groups. Lesions are bilateral and started posteriorly.

19.5 Histological Features

Dabska and Buraczewski [11] observed that the excised part of the bone looked like an inflated balloon with raised periosteum. Immediately underneath the periosteum, a thin osseous shell was present and covered the entire tumor. Under the shell the bone was completely destroyed and replaced by a labyrinth of rounded cavities of various sizes filled with large quantities of liquid blood (Figs. 19.2, 19.3, and 19.4).

On section aneurysmal bone cyst presents the appearance of a cavernous vascular tumor. In long bones the eccentric localization is evident. The cavities are surrounded by whitish-gray or brownish elastic fibrous tissue. The diameter of the cavities is from a few mm to 1 or 2 cm. The inner surfaces are smooth and glossy. The cavities are intercommunicating and do not contain clots. In some cases, structural differences may appear. Some tumors have a strikingly cystic character with

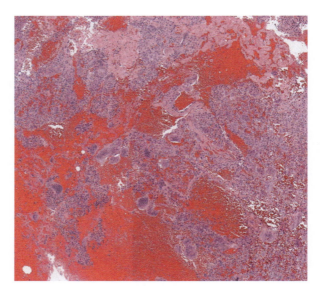

Fig. 19.2 Image 4×

19.5 Histological Features

Fig. 19.3 Image 10×

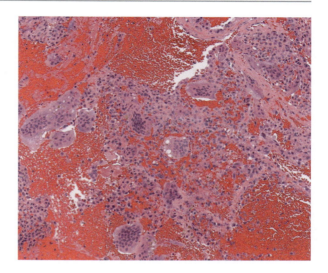

Fig. 19.4 Image 40×

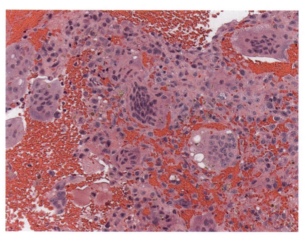

multiple small cysts divided by scanty fibrous connective tissue. On section some tumors resemble a sponge, while others are more fibrous with fewer cavities and look like Swiss cheese. In the fibrous tissue dividing the cavities, some osseous elements may be seen even with the naked eye.

Microscopic features may differ in detail from case to case. In the resected tumor, the most striking picture is the presence of multiple large and small cavities of various sizes, some swollen and filled with blood, others empty with loose walls or filled with packed proteinaceous material. No tumor has endothelial lining or smooth muscle tissue in the walls of dilated muscular spaces. However, in some tumors many bulging vessels are present, mostly capillaries, and give the impression of being under blood pressure.

These vessels and vascular spaces are supported by connective tissue with filamentous trabeculae of newly formed bone. Around the spaces varying numbers of multinuclear giant cells are present. Sometimes they cause the diagnostic error of giant cell tumors. It should be remembered that giant cell tumors (unless irradiated) do not produce osteoid. The presence of osteoid tissue and of bony trabeculae may be taken as evidence against a diagnosis of osteoclastoma. Moreover, the affected bone area, which is composed mostly of blood-filled cavities, is covered by the periosteum and outlined by a thin subperiosteal bone shell. The latter feature, although not exclusive to aneurysmal bone cyst, is a constant finding.

In some of the solid areas, sheets of vascular tissue, containing large numbers of multinucleated giant cells, fibroblast, hemorrhage, and hemosiderin, look very much like giant cell granuloma of the jaws. Other solid areas may have the appearance of fibrous dysplasia, ossifying fibroma, and possibly other jaw tumors. This gives evidence to the view that the aneurysmal bone cyst may represent secondary changes in pre-existing lesion.

According to Clough and Price [2], there are no cellular features suggestive of malignant neoplasia unless, of course, the cyst has developed in a malignant tumor.

Liu et al. [12] undertook a comparison of the histopathology of giant cell lesions of the jaws and concluded that aneurysmal bone cyst is primarily a giant cell lesion and is related to giant cell granuloma of the jaws.

19.6 Treatment

The mainstay of treatment is surgery. The majority of patients undergo curettage, bone graft, and/or cementation.

References

1. Jaffe HL, Lichtenstein L. Solitary unicameral bone cyst with emphasis on the Roentgen picture, the pathologic appearance, and the pathogenesis. Arch Surg. 1942;44:1004–25.
2. Clough JR, Price CHG. Aneurysmal bone cysts. J Bone Joint Surg Br. 1968;50:110–27.
3. Bernier JL, Bhaskar SN. Aneurysmal bone cysts of the mandible. Oral Surg Oral Med Oral Pathol. 1958;11:1018–28.
4. Kransdorf MJ, Sweet DE. Aneurysmal bone cyst: concept, controversy, clinical presentation, and imaging. AJR Am J Roentgenol. 1995;164:573–80.
5. Struthers PJ, Shear M. Aneurysmal bone cyst of the jaws. (II). Pathogenesis. Int J Oral Surg. 1984;13:92–100.
6. Geschickter CF, Copeland M. Tumors of bone. 3rd ed. Philadelphia: J.B. Lippincott; 1949.
7. Jaffe HL. Giant cell reparative granuloma, traumatic bone cyst and fibrous (fibro-osseous) dysplasia of the jawbones. Oral Surg Oral Med Oral Pathol. 1953;6:159–75.
8. Fisher AD. Bone cavities in fibro-osseous lesions. Br J Oral Surg. 1976;14:120–7.
9. Struthers PJ, Shear M. Aneurysmal bone cyst of the jaws. (I) Clinicopathological features. Int J Oral Surg. 1984;13:85–9.
10. Levy WM, Miller AS, Bonakdarpour A, Aegerter E. Aneurysmal bone cyst secondary to other osseous lesions. Report of 57 cases. Am J Clin Pathol. 1975;63:1–8.
11. Dabska M, Buraczewski J. Aneurysmal bone cyst: pathology, clinical course and radiologic appearances. Cancer. 1969;23:371–89.
12. Liu B, Yu SF, Li TJ. Multinucleated giant cells in various forms of giant cell containing lesions of the jaws express features of osteoclasts. J Oral Pathol Med. 2003;32:367–75.

Calcifying Odontogenic Cyst

Calcifying Cystic Odontogenic Tumor

20

Contents

20.1	Suggested Classification of the Odontogenic Ghost Cell Lesions	84
20.2	Pathogenesis	84
20.3	Clinical Features	85
20.4	Radiological Features	85
20.5	Differential Diagnosis	86
20.6	Histological Features	86
20.7	Treatment	88
References		88

The term calcifying odontogenic cyst (COC) was first introduced by Gorlin and his colleagues [1]. The COC is a developmental odontogenic cyst with diverse origin as either a cyst or a neoplasm.

Calcifying odontogenic cyst was earlier thought to be an oral presentation of cutaneous calcifying epithelioma of Malherbe (1982). It was also termed as "*keratinizing cyst*" and referred to as a cyst by Chen and Miller. Gold found keratinization as a prominent feature and therefore renamed the lesion as "*keratinizing and calcifying odontogenic cyst*" (KCOC). Because of the varied histopathologic characteristics, various terminologies have been proposed which include "*calcifying ghost cell odontogenic tumor*" (CGCOT) proposed by Fejerskov and Krogh [2] and "*cystic calcifying odontogenic tumor*" (CCOT) proposed by Freedman et al. [3].

The studies of Praetorius et al. [4] led WHO to conclude that what had previously been regarded as a calcifying odontogenic cyst actually comprised two entities: a cyst and a neoplasm. In the latest WHO publication on odontogenic tumors [5], it was classified as a benign odontogenic tumor and was renamed "*calcifying cystic odontogenic tumor*" (CCOT).

© The Author(s), under exclusive license to Springer Nature Singapore Pte Ltd. 2024
K. Paiwal et al., *Handbook of Oral and Maxillofacial Giant Cell Lesions*,
https://doi.org/10.1007/978-981-97-2863-3_20

20.1 Suggested Classification of the Odontogenic Ghost Cell Lesions

(From Praetorius 2006, personal communication)

- Group 1
  - "Simple" cysts
  - Calcifying odontogenic cyst (COC)
- Group 2
- Cysts associated with odontogenic hamartomas or benign neoplasms: calcifying cystic odontogenic tumors (CCOT). The following combinations have been published:
  - CCOT associated with an odontoma
  - CCOT associated with AOT; CCOT associated with ameloblastoma
  - CCOT associated with ameloblastic fibroma
  - CCOT associated with ameloblastic fibro-odontoma; CCOT associated with odontoameloblastoma
  - CCOT associated with odontogenic myxofibroma
- Group 3
- Solid benign odontogenic neoplasms with similar cell morphology to that in the COC and with dentinoid formation
  - Dentinogenic ghost cell tumor
- Group 4
- Malignant odontogenic neoplasms with features similar to those of the dentinogenic ghost cell tumor
  - Ghost cell odontogenic carcinoma

20.2 Pathogenesis

The pathogenesis is considerably complicated by the fact that the epithelial lining of a calcifying odontogenic cyst appears to have the ability to induce the formation of dental tissues in the adjacent connective tissue wall and that other odontogenic tumors such as the ameloblastoma, the odontoameloblastoma, the ameloblastic fibroma, and the ameloblastic fibro-odontoma may sometimes be associated with it [6–10].

Takeda et al. [11] was convinced that the cysts arise de novo, as were Praetorius et al. [4], who concluded from their study that substantial evidence existed that the tumor developed from the wall of the cyst. They suggested that the calcifying odontogenic cyst was a unicystic process that developed from reduced enamel epithelium or remnants of odontogenic epithelium in the follicle, gingival tissue, or bone. Dentinoid alone or an odontome may be found in the cyst wall, induced by the lining epithelium. Praetorius believes that the dentinogenic ghost cell tumor is a neoplasm de novo, but the COC plus benign neoplasm or hamartoma is a cyst from the beginning.

20.3 Clinical Features

The terms used for the solid neoplastic variant of COC were *"dentinogenic ghost cell tumor"* (DGCT) by Praetorius et al., *"epithelial odontogenic ghost cell tumor"* (EOGCT) by Ellis and Shmookler [12], *"odontogenic ghost cell tumor"* (OGCT) by Colmenero et al. [13], and *"odontogenic ghost cell ameloblastoma"* by Shear [14]. The lesion accounts for 1% of all odontogenic jaw cysts. The cystic or nonneoplastic variant of COC is found to occur in 80–98% of cases and is associated with odontoma in 24% of cases. The solid or neoplastic variant of COC accounted for about 11.5% of cases. The COC are usually intraosseous (70% of the cases) with extraosseous presentation accounting for 16–22% mostly seen in individuals above the age of 50 years.

The age ranges from 1 to 82 years with peak in the second decade. In their study Praetorius et al. [4] and Buchner [15] have drawn attention to bimodal age distribution with peaks in the second and sixth decades.

The lesion has no sex predilection as well as is equally distributed between the maxilla and mandible. COC are common anterior to the first molar region in which 75% of cases are in the incisor canine region or inter-canine region usually crossing the midline of the mandible, which is a rare feature in the maxilla.

Swelling is the most frequent complaint and has occurred in about half of the reported cases. Only rarely has there been pain. Intraosseous lesions may produce a hard bony expansion and may be fairly extensive. Lingual expansion may sometimes be observed. Occasionally, the calcifying odontogenic cyst may perforate the cortical plate and extend into the soft tissues. In a few cases, displacement of the teeth has been described. Extraosseous lesions tend to be pink to red, circumscribed elevated masses measuring up to 4 cm in diameter.

20.4 Radiological Features

The intraosseous variant of COC presents as a well-defined radiolucent entity with internal calcifications varying from small flecks to large masses. Usually unilocular, the lesion can occur pericoronal to impacted tooth (Fig. 20.1). Rarely, they may be multilocular. The margins are well-corticated and may be expansile. Displacement of teeth and resorption of the roots of adjacent teeth are frequent findings. The extraosseous lesions show localized superficial bone resorption or saucer-shaped radiolucencies and sometimes displace adjacent teeth.

Below is the reconstructed panoramic view of a case of COC. Note the well-defined, unilocular, pericoronal radiolucent lesion associated with impacted right mandibular third molar (yellow arrow). Flecks of radiopacities are seen within the radiolucency (orange arrows).

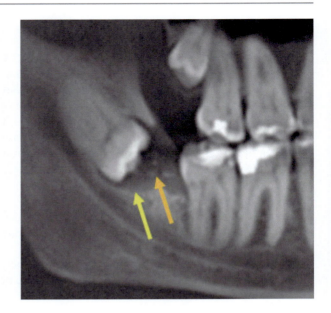

Fig. 20.1 CBCT custom-made section. Note the well-defined, unilocular, pericoronal radiolucent lesion associated with impacted right mandibular third molar (yellow arrow). Flecks of radiopacities are seen within the radiolucency (orange arrow)

20.5　Differential Diagnosis

1. **Adenomatoid odontogenic tumor**: Occurs in younger age group, predominantly female and in anterior maxilla.
2. **Calcifying epithelial odontogenic cyst**: More common in younger age groups, occurs anterior to the first molar.
3. **Ameloblastic fibro-odontoma**: More common in younger age groups and in the first molar region.
4. **Mural ameloblastoma**: Occurs usually in younger patients; expansion and tooth displacement are more prominent. No radiopaque foci are associated with the lesion.
5. **Dentigerous cysts**: Unilocular radiolucent entity attached to CEJ of the involved tooth. No evidence of internal calcification except in old standing cyst.

20.6　Histological Features

The epithelial lining has characteristic odontogenic features with a prominent basal layer consisting of palisaded columnar or cuboidal cells and hyperchromatic nuclei which are polarized away from the basement membrane. The epithelium may be regular six to eight cells thick over part of its length and be continuous with parts that may be very thin and others that are considerably thickened. Budding from the basal layer into the adjacent connective tissue and epithelial proliferations into the lumen are frequently seen (Figs. 20.2, 20.3, and 20.4).

20.6 Histological Features

Fig. 20.2 Image 4×

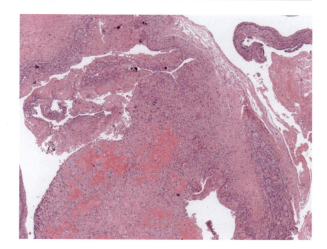

Fig. 20.3 Image 10×

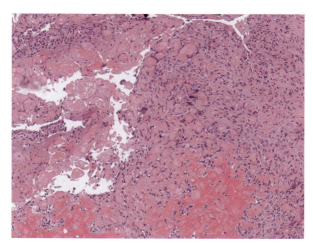

Fig. 20.4 Image 40×

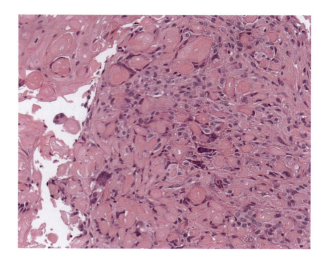

The most remarkable feature of the COC is the presence of ghost cells. The ghost cells are found in groups, particularly in the thicker areas of the epithelial lining. The spinous cells in such situations may be widely separated by intercellular edema and the epithelium around the ghost cells is often convoluted.

The ghost cells are enlarged, ballooned, and ovoid or elongated ellipsoid epithelial cells. They are eosinophilic and although the cell outlines are usually well-defined, they may sometimes be blurred so that groups of them appear fused. A few ghost cells may contain nuclear remnants, but these are in various stages of degeneration, and in the majority all traces of chromatin have disappeared leaving only a faint outline of the original nucleus. The ghost cells represent an abnormal type of keratinization and have an affinity for calcification. Ghost cells may represent the products of coagulative necrosis of odontogenic epithelium. Sapp and Gardner [16] found that calcification may occur in some of the ghost cells, and ultrastructural studies have shown to represent dystrophic calcification.

The ghost cells may be in contact with the connective tissue wall of the cyst where they may then evoke a foreign body reaction with the formation of multinucleated giant cells. In the fibrous wall, there are usually strands and islands of odontogenic epithelium, either in direct contact with the epithelium or separately in the connective tissue. An atubular dentinoid is often found in the wall close to the epithelial lining and often in relation to the epithelial proliferations. It is found particularly in contact with masses of ghost cells.

20.7 Treatment

The COC is treated by surgical enucleation unless it is associated with another odontogenic tumor, in which case wider excision may be required.

References

1. Gorlin RJ, Pindborg JJ, Clausen FP, Vickers RA. The calcifying odontogenic cyst—A possible analogue of the cutaneous calcifying epithelioma of Malherbe. An analysis of fifteen cases. Oral Surg Oral Med Oral Pathol. 1962;15:1235–43.
2. Fejerskov O, Krogh J. The calcifying ghost cell odontogenic tumor: or the calcifying odontogenic cyst. J Oral Pathol. 1972;1:273–87.
3. Freedman PD, Lumerman H, Gee JK. Calcifying odontogenic cyst. Oral Surg Oral Med Oral Pathol. 1975;40:93–106.
4. Prætorius F, Hjørting-Hansen E, Gorlin RJ, Vickers RA. Calcifying odontogenic cyst. Range, variations and neoplastic potential. Acta Odontol Scand. 1981;39:227–40.
5. Prætorius F, Ledesma-Montes C. Calcifying cystic odontogenic tumor. In: Barnes L, Eveson JW, Reichart P, Sidransky D, editors. Pathology and genetics. Head and neck tumors. Lyon: World Health Organization Classification of Tumors, IARC Press; 2005. p. 313.
6. Prætorius F. Calcifying odontogenic cyst: range, variations and neoplastic potential. Paper delivered at a symposium on maxillofacial bone pathology, Brussels, 30–31 March 1974, organized by Committee on Maxillofacial Bone Pathology. Int J Oral Surg. 1975;4:89 (Abstract).

References

7. Hirshberg A, Kaplan I, Buchner A. Calcifying odontogenic cyst associated with odontoma: a possible separate entity (odontocalcifying odontogenic cyst). J Oral Maxillofac Surg. 1994;52:555–8.
8. Aithal D, Reddy BS, Mahajan S, Boaz K, Kamboj M. Ameloblastomatous calcifying odontogenic cyst: a rare histologic variant. J Oral Pathol Med. 2003;32:376–8.
9. Lin CC, Chen CH, Lin LM, et al. Oral surgery. Oral Med Oral Pathol Oral Radiol Endod. 2004;98:451–60.
10. Iida S, Ueda T, Aikawa T, et al. Ameloblastomatous calcifying odontogenic cyst in the mandible. Dentomaxillofac Radiol. 2004;33:409–12.
11. Takeda Y, Suzuki A, Yamamoto H. Histopathologic study of epithelial components in the connective tissue wall of unilocular type of calcifying odontogenic cyst. J Oral Pathol Med. 1990;19:108–13.
12. https://www.sciencedirect.com/science/article/abs/pii/0030422086903907.
13. Colmenero C, Patron M, Colmenero B. Odontogenic ghost cell tumors. J Craniomaxillofac Surg. 1990;18:215–8.
14. Shear M. Developmental odontogenic cysts. An update. J Oral Pathol Med. 1994;23:1–11.
15. Buchner A. The central (intraosseous) calcifying odontogenic cyst: an analysis of 215 cases. J Oral Maxillofac Surg. 1991;49:330–9.
16. Sapp JP, Gardner DG. An ultrastructural study of the calcifications in calcifying odontogenic cysts and odontomas. Oral Surg Oral Med Oral Pathol. 1977;44:754–66.

Resorption of Teeth

21

Contents

21.1 Physiological Condition.. 91
21.2 Histology of Shedding... 92
21.3 Nonphysiological Conditions.. 92
     21.3.1 External Resorption.. 93
     21.3.2 Internal Resorption... 98
21.4 Treatment and Prognosis.. 100
References.. 100

21.1 Physiological Condition

The exfoliation of deciduous teeth is a physiologic phenomenon and results in the elimination of the deciduous dentition.

The permanent incisors and canines develop lingually to the deciduous teeth and erupt in an occlusal and vestibular direction. Resorption of deciduous tooth roots occurs on the lingual surface and these teeth are shed with much of their pulp chamber intact. Permanent premolars develop between the divergent roots of deciduous molars and erupt in an occlusal direction. Hence, the resorption of interradicular dentin takes place with some resorption of the pulp chamber, coronal dentin, and sometimes enamel.

© The Author(s), under exclusive license to Springer Nature Singapore Pte
Ltd. 2024
K. Paiwal et al., *Handbook of Oral and Maxillofacial Giant Cell Lesions*,
https://doi.org/10.1007/978-981-97-2863-3_21

21.2   Histology of Shedding

The cells responsible for the removal of dental hard tissue are identical to osteoclasts and are called odontoclasts. Odontoclasts are readily identifiable in the light microscope as large, multinucleated cells occupying resorption bays on the surface of a dental hard tissue. Their cytoplasm is vacuolated and the surface of the cell adjacent to the resorbing hard tissue forms a "brush" border. The brush border is resolved as a ruffled border produced by extensive folding of the cell membrane into a series of invaginations 2–3 μm deep, with mineral crystallites within the depth of the invaginations. The cytoplasm of the odontoclast is characterized by an exceptionally high content of mitochondria and many vacuoles, which are especially concentrated adjacent to the ruffled border. Acid phosphatase activity occurs within these vacuoles. Histochemically, a characteristic feature of the odontoclast is a high level of activity of the enzyme acid phosphatase.

Odontoclasts probably have the same origin as osteoclasts. Odontoclasts are derived from the monocyte and migrate from blood vessels to the resorption site, where they fuse to form the characteristic multinucleated odontoclast with a clear attachment zone and ruffled border.

Odontoclasts are most commonly found on surfaces of the roots in relation to the advancing permanent tooth. When root resorption is almost complete, the odontoblasts degenerate, and mononuclear cells emerge from pulpal vessels and migrate to the predentin surface, where they fuse with other mononuclear cells to form odontoclasts actively engaged in the removal of predentin and dentin. Just before exfoliation, resorption ceases as the odontoclasts migrate away from the dentin surface and the remaining pulp cells now deposit cement like tissue on it. The tooth then sheds, with some pulpal tissue intact. During this process, odontoclasts resorb unmineralized dentin.

21.3   Nonphysiological Conditions

Resorption in permanent teeth will occur only under pathologic conditions. This fact appears to be due to the anti-resorptive properties of the precementum covering of the root that protects it in the presence of inflammation.

Since resorption of a tooth may begin either on the external surface (arising due to tissue reaction in the periodontal or pericoronal tissue) or inside the tooth (from a pulpal tissue reaction), the general terms "external resorption" and "internal resorption" are used to distinguish between the two types. The chief causes or situations in which resorption may occur are as follows:

1. External resorption
   (a) Periapical inflammation
   (b) Reimplantation of teeth
   (c) Tumors and cysts

21.3 Nonphysiological Conditions

    (d) Excessive mechanical or occlusal forces
    (e) Impaction of teeth
    (f) Idiopathic
2. Internal resorption
    (a) Idiopathic

21.3.1 External Resorption

21.3.1.1 Resorption Associated with Periapical Inflammation

Resorption of calcified dental tissues occurs in the same fashion as that of bone and may or may not be associated with the presence of osteoclasts.

A periapical granuloma arising as a result of pulpal infection or trauma occasionally causes subsequent resorption of the root apex if the inflammatory lesion persists for a sufficient period of time. Most teeth involved by a periapical granuloma, however, do not exhibit any significant degree of resorption. The reason for the occasional occurrence is not known. The bone is more readily resorbed than dental tissue as borne out by the fact that bone is always destroyed when a periapical granuloma develops, whereas resorption of the tooth root without loss of bone seldom occurs except at a microscopic level.

21.3.1.2 Radiographic Features

Even though it can occur in any tooth surface, the common areas for external root resorption are apical and cervical regions (Figs. 21.1, 21.2, and 21.3). In the case of apical resorption, it appears as slight raggedness or blunting of the root apex in the early stages, proceeding to a severe loss of tooth substance. Lamina dura and periodontal ligament space around the tooth will be intact. When the condition is associated with periapical inflammation, the lamina will be lost along with widening of the apical periodontal ligament space.

21.3.1.3 Differential Diagnosis

1. **Caries**: Located always above the level of the interdental alveolar bone.
2. **Internal resorption**: Expansion of the pulp chamber or canal is characteristic for internal resorption. Making two radiographs with slightly differing horizontal angulation (tube shift technique) may help in differentiating the lesions.

21.3.1.4 Reimplanted Teeth

The reimplantation or transplantation of teeth almost invariably results in severe resorption of the root. The tooth substance must be considered non-vital tissue. Thus, the implanted tooth is analogous to a bone graft which acts only as a temporary scaffold and is ultimately resorbed and replaced.

If the tooth remains outside of the socket without being placed in a proper storage medium, then the PDL cells will undergo necrosis. Without vital PDL cells, the surrounding bone will view the tooth as a foreign object and initiate resorption and replacement by bone.

Fig. 21.1 Mandibular anterior periapical radiographs showing a radiolucency superimposed over the right mandibular central incisor (yellow arrow). Note the absence of enlargement of the root canal

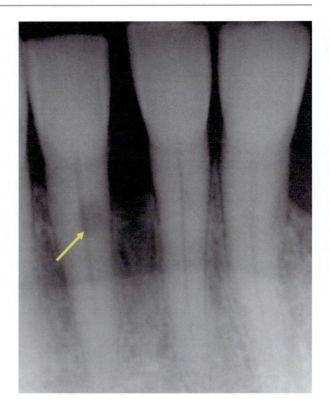

The tooth root is resorbed and replaced by bone, producing an ankylosis. If the tooth root does not become completely resorbed, the ensuing ankylosis may result in a functional tooth. Many reimplanted teeth, however, exhibit complete resorption of the root and are exfoliated.

21.3.1.5 Tumors and Cysts

Both benign and malignant tumors may cause root resorption, although benign lesions are more likely to produce displacement than actual destruction of the tooth (Fig. 21.4). In most cases connective tissue is present between the tumor and the tooth, and it is from this tissue that cells develop, chiefly osteoclasts, which appear to be responsible for the root resorption.

Cysts cause root resorption in a manner similar to resorption caused by benign tumors, that is, chiefly by pressure, although displacement of the tooth is more common than resorption.

21.3.1.6 Excessive Mechanical or Occlusal Forces

The usual form of excessive mechanical force with which root resorption may be associated is that applied during orthodontic treatment (Fig. 21.5).

21.3 Nonphysiological Conditions

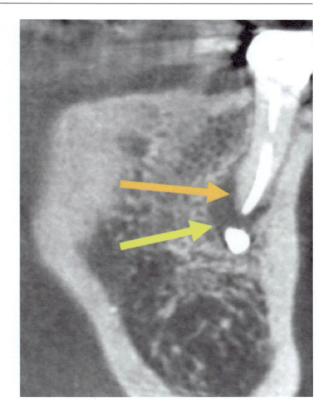

Fig. 21.2 CBCT sagittal section of endodontically treated mandibular first premolar showing external root resorption. Note the blunting and raggedness of the root apex along (orange arrow) with periapical rarefying osteitis (yellow arrow). The gutta-percha is seen extruding from the apex along with extruded radiopaque sealant material

Becks reported that systemic disturbances, mainly hypothyroidism, may predispose to root resorption, particularly in the patient receiving orthodontic treatment. However, the influence of systemic factor remains to be confirmed.

The bone undergoes resorption far more readily than cementum when force is exerted upon the tooth by orthodontic appliances or by occlusal trauma. Small lacunae often appear on the surface of the cementum and ultimately extend into the dentin, indicating early tooth resorption. Probably most cases of this minor type of resorption are soon repaired by the deposition of bone or cementum in these ragged lacunae, particularly if the occlusal force or orthodontic pressure is relieved.

From a histological point of view, different degrees of orthodontically induced inflammatory root resorption severity are determined by the extent to which root tissue is involved. On that basis, three different types of orthodontically induced inflammatory root resorption can be distinguished.

– **Surface resorption**: In this process, only the outer cemental layers are resorbed, and they are fully regenerated or remodeled once the etiological factor has been removed.

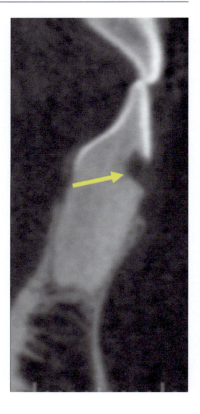

Fig. 21.3 CBCT sagittal section showing invasive cervical resorption in mandibular anterior tooth. Note the cervical radiolucency on the labial aspect extending toward the pulp chamber but not involving it (yellow arrow)

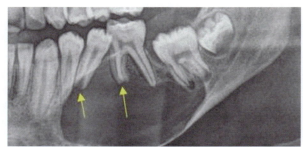

Fig. 21.4 Cropped panoramic radiographs showing a large cyst in the left mandibular region causing resorption of the mesial root of mandibular first molar and both the premolars (yellow arrows). (Courtesy A.Z. Syed, BDS, MHA, MS, Dipl. ABOMR)

- **Deep resorption**: In this process, the cementum and the outer layers of dentin are resorbed and usually repaired with cementum material. The final shape of the root after this resorption and formation process may or may not be identical to the original form.
- **Circumferential apical root resorption**: In this process, tridimensional resorption of the hard tissue components of the root apex occurs, and root shortening is evident.

21.3 Nonphysiological Conditions

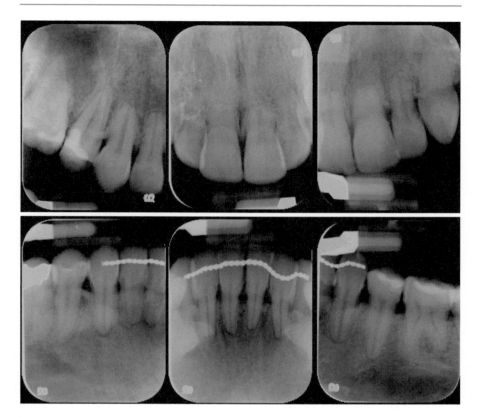

Fig. 21.5 Periapical radiographs of a post-orthodontic case showing generalized apical root resorption

21.3.1.7 Impacted Teeth

Teeth that are completely impacted or embedded in bone occasionally will undergo resorption of the crown or of both crown and root. Stafne and Austin reported that teeth that are completely embedded are those most apt to undergo resorption. In a study of 226 embedded teeth in which resorption occurred, they found that 78% of the teeth were in the maxillary arch and that 60% of these maxillary teeth were cuspids. Thus, although maxillary and mandibular third molars far outnumber maxillary cuspids in incidence of impaction, the cuspids undergo resorption more frequently than the third molars. The reason for this is unknown. Impacted supernumerary teeth, particularly mesiodens, also are prone to undergo resorption.

Impacted teeth also may cause resorption of the roots of adjacent teeth without being resorbed themselves (Fig. 21.6). This is particularly common in the case of a horizontally or mesioangularly impacted mandibular third molar impinging on the roots of the second molar.

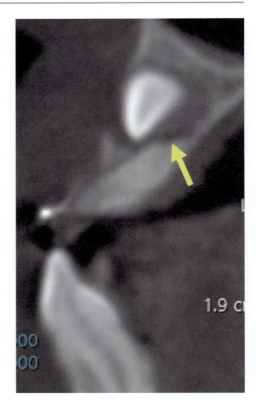

Fig. 21.6 CBCT sagittal section showing impacted maxillary canine causing root resorption of the adjacent tooth (yellow arrow)

21.3.1.8 Idiopathic Resorption

Many investigators have reported that the roots of permanent teeth may undergo a certain amount of resorption in apparently normal adults without any obvious cause.

Massler and Perreault [1] in their study observed that the teeth most commonly involved by root resorption were the maxillary bicuspids, while the mandibular incisors and molars exhibited the least resorption.

A rare form of multiple idiopathic root resorptions may occur that involves all or nearly all of the teeth. The resorption may begin at the cementoenamel junction or nearer to the root apex. This disease has been discussed by Kerr and his associates who pointed out that these patients are medically normal and have no past history such as orthodontic treatment or radiation that might explain the phenomenon.

21.3.2 Internal Resorption

21.3.2.1 Chronic Perforating Hyperplasia of the Pulp, Internal Granuloma, Odontoclastoma, Pink Tooth of Mummery

Internal resorption is a relatively rare occurrence and most cases follow injury to pulpal tissues, such as physical trauma or caries-related pulpitis. The resorption can continue as long as vital pulp tissue remains and may result in communication of the pulp with the periodontal ligament.

21.3 Nonphysiological Conditions

Sweet [2] has presented a historic review of the internal resorption of teeth, beginning with the first description of the problem.

21.3.2.2 Clinical Features

Most cases of internal resorption present no early clinical symptoms. The first evidence of the lesion may be the appearance of a pink-hued area on the crown of the tooth, which represents the hyperplastic, vascular pulp tissue filling the resorbed area and showing through the remaining overlying tooth substance.

21.3.2.3 Radiographic Features

The involved tooth exhibits a round or ovoid radiolucent area in the central portion of the tooth, continuous with the pulp but not with the external surface of the tooth unless the condition is of such duration that perforation has occurred (Fig. 21.7). The pulp chamber appears enlarged.

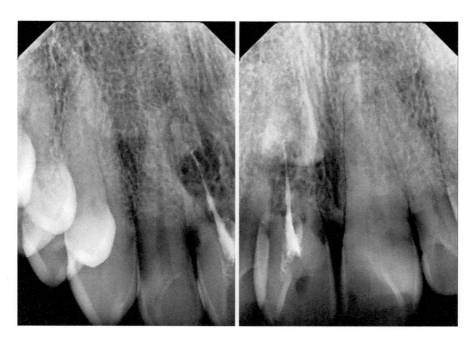

Fig. 21.7 Periapical radiographs showing internal root resorption involving right maxillary central incisor causing loss of almost the entire tooth along with perforation

21.3.2.4 Differential Diagnosis

Depending on the resorption location sometimes, this resorption is easily visualized with imaging.

1. **Caries**: Located always above the level of the interdental alveolar bone.
2. **External resorption**: Normal intact pulp chamber or canal. However, this may be difficult to detect radiographically. Making two radiographs with slightly differing horizontal angulation (tube shift technique) may help in differentiating the lesions.

21.3.2.5 Histological Features

Two main patterns are seen: (1) inflammatory resorption and (2) replacement or metaplastic absorption. In inflammatory resorption, the resorbed dentin is replaced by inflamed granulation tissue. The resorption continues as long as vital pulp remains. In this pattern the area of destruction usually appears as a uniform, well-circumscribed symmetric radiolucent enlargement of the pulp chamber or canal. In replacement resorption, portions of the pulpal dentinal walls are resorbed and replaced with bone or cementum-like bone.

In patients with internal inflammatory resorption, the pulp tissue in the area of destruction is vascular and exhibits increased cellularity and collagenization. Immediately adjacent to the dentinal wall are numerous multinucleated dentinoclasts, which are histologically and functionally identical to osteoclasts. An inflammatory infiltrate characterized by lymphocytes, histiocytes, and polymorphonuclear leukocytes is not uncommon.

In replacement resorption, the normal pulp tissue is replaced by woven bone that fuses with the adjacent dentin.

21.4 Treatment and Prognosis

The treatment of internal and external resorption centers on the removal of all soft tissue from the sites of dental destruction.

References

1. Massler M, Perreault JG. Root resorption in the permanent teeth of young adults. J Dent Child. 1954;21:158.
2. Sweet APS. Internal resorption. A chronology. Dent Radiogr Photogr. 1965;38:75.

Tuberculosis

22

Contents

22.1   Etiology.. 102
22.2   Pathogenesis.. 102
22.3   Clinical Features.. 102
22.4   Route of Infection.. 103
22.5   Laboratory Diagnosis.. 104
22.6   Oral Manifestations.. 105
22.7   Tuberculous Osteomyelitis of Jaws.................................. 105
22.8   Scrofula.. 106
22.9   Histopathology... 106
22.10 Diagnosis... 107
22.11 Treatment.. 108
Reference.. 108

Tuberculosis is a specific infectious granulomatous disease caused by *Mycobacterium tuberculosis*. *M. tuberculosis* infects about one third of the world's population and is the single most important cause of death on Earth by infection. It commonly affects lungs but also affects the intestines, meninges, bones, joints, lymph glands, skin, and other tissues of the body. The disease also affects animals like cattle; this is known as bovine tuberculosis and is sometimes communicated to man through ingestion of unpasteurized, infected cow's milk.

Hansen (1968) identified the lepra bacillus, the first member of this genus. Koch (1882) isolated the mammalian tubercle bacillus and proved its causative role in tuberculosis by satisfying Koch's postulates. Johne (1895) described *Mycobacterium paratuberculosis*, the agent causing chronic specific entities in cattle [1].

© The Author(s), under exclusive license to Springer Nature Singapore Pte Ltd. 2024
K. Paiwal et al., *Handbook of Oral and Maxillofacial Giant Cell Lesions*,
https://doi.org/10.1007/978-981-97-2863-3_22

22.1 Etiology

Two species of *Mycobacterium* cause tuberculosis: *M. tuberculosis* and *M. bovis*. *M. tuberculosis* is transmitted by inhalation of infective droplets, coughed or sneezed into the air by a patient with tuberculosis. *M. bovis* is transmitted by milk from diseased cows.

M. avium and *M. intracellulare*, two closely related mycobacteria, have no virulence in normal hosts but cause disseminated infections in 15–24% of patients with AIDS. Mycobacteria are aerobic, rod-shaped, nonspore-forming, acid-fast bacilli.

22.2 Pathogenesis

The pathogenicity of *M. tuberculosis* is related to its ability to escape killing by macrophages and induce delayed-type hypersensitivity. This has been attributed to several components of bacterial cell wall.

1. The cord factor, a surface glycolipid that causes *M. tuberculosis* to grow in serpentine cords.
2. The sulfatides, which are surface glycolipids containing sulfur and prevent fusion of phagosomes of macrophages containing *M. tuberculosis* with the lysosomes.
3. LAM, a major heteropolysaccharide, inhibits macrophage activation by interferon gamma. It induces macrophages to secrete TNF-α, which causes fever, weight loss, and tissue damage, as well as IL-10, which suppresses T-cell proliferation.
4. *M. tuberculosis* heat-shock protein induces autoimmune reaction.

The development of cell-mediated or type IV hypersensitivity to the tubercle bacillus probably explains the organism's destructiveness in tissues and also the emergence of resistance to the organisms. On the initial exposure to the organism, a nonspecific inflammatory response develops. Within 2 or 3 weeks, the reaction becomes granulomatous and the centers of granulomas become caseous, forming typical "soft tubercles." The pattern of host response depends on whether the infection represents a primary exposure or secondary reaction.

22.3 Clinical Features

Primary tuberculosis is usually asymptomatic. Occasionally, fever and pleural effusion may occur.

Classically, the lesions of secondary tuberculosis are located in the apex of the lungs but may spread to many different sites by expectorated infected material or through the lymphatic and vascular channels. Typically, patients have a low-grade fever, malaise, anorexia, weight loss, and night sweats. With pulmonary progression, a productive cough develops, often with hemoptysis or chest pain. Any organ system may be involved, including the lymphatic system, skin, skeletal system, central nervous system, kidneys, and gastrointestinal tract. Involvement of the skin has been called lupus vulgaris.

Head and neck involvement is not rare. The most common extrapulmonary sites in head and neck are the cervical lymph nodes followed by the larynx and middle ear. Much fewer common sites include the nasal cavity, nasopharynx, oral cavity, parotid gland, esophagus, and spine.

22.4 Route of Infection

There are three routes of primary infection.

- Direct spread to lungs
- From tonsil to the lymph node of the neck, where an abscess may form and track round the edge of the sternomastoid muscle producing collar stud abscess
- From lower ileal infection to the lymph nodes of ileocecal angle

With the primary involvement of the lungs, commonly seen in children, the alveolar macrophages engulf the bacilli, multiply, and produce a subpleural focus of tuberculous pneumonia, commonly located in the lower lobe or the lower part of the upper lobe (Ghon's focus). The Ghon's focus together with the enlarged hilar lymph node is called the "primary complex." This occurs about 3–8 weeks, from the time of infection, and is associated with a development of tuberculin hypersensitivity. In most cases, the healing of the lesion occurs spontaneously in 2–6 months leaving behind a calcified nodule. However, a few bacilli may survive in the healed lesion and remain latent.

In children with impaired immunity or other risk factors, the primary lesion may enlarge and cause miliary, meningeal, or other forms of disseminated tuberculosis. The seeding can take place to any organ in the body.

The post-primary type (secondary tuberculosis) is due to reactivation of latent infections or exogenous reinfection. It affects mainly the upper lobe of the lungs; the lesion goes under necrosis and tissue destruction, leading to cavitation. The necrotic materials break into the airways, leading to expectoration of bacteria-laden sputum, which is the main source of infection to contacts.

Depending on the time of infection and type of response, tuberculosis may be classified as "primary" and "post-primary" or "secondary."

Primary Tuberculosis

It is the form of disease that develops in a previously unexposed and therefore desensitized person. The commonly affected are elderly because of waning immunity and immunosuppressed individuals as in those with AIDS. The disease may develop without any interruption into the so-called progressive primary tuberculosis, commonly seen in HIV-positive patients with an advanced degree of immunosuppression (i.e., CD4+ counts <200 cells/mm^3).

Primary infection may either extend locally or become disseminated or more commonly undergo progressive fibrosis, often followed by radiologically detectable calcification (Ranke complex).

Secondary Tuberculosis

It arises in a previously sensitized host. It may follow shortly after primary infection but commonly arises from reactivation of the dormant primary lesion when the host defense is weakened. It may also result from exogenous reinfection or reactivation of endogenous lesions. Only a few patients (>5%) develop secondary tuberculosis.

Secondary pulmonary tuberculosis is classically localized to the apex of one or both upper lobes which may relate to the high oxygen tension in the apices. Cavitations occur readily resulting along the airways.

22.5   Laboratory Diagnosis

Blood investigations/hematology

1. Complete hemogram
   (a) Monocytosis (8–10%)
   (b) Elevated ESR
   (c) Anemia

   Microscopy

1. Smear staining

Samples can be obtained from sputum, urine, body fluids, or tissues of the patient and smears prepared. Tuberculous bacilli are stained using Ziehl-Neelsen staining technique as given below:

1. The smear is covered with strong carbol fuchsin and gently heated to steaming for 5–7 mins, without letting the stain boil and become dry.
2. The slide is then washed with water and decolorized with 20% sulfuric acid till no color comes off and then washed with 95% ethanol for 2 min.
3. The smear is counterstained with Loeffler's methylene blue 1%.

22.6 Oral Manifestations

Oral lesions of tuberculosis are uncommon. Oral manifestations that usually follow implantation of *M. tuberculosis* from infected sputum may appear on any mucosal surface. The tongue and the palate are favored locations. The typical lesion is an indurated, chronic, nonhealing ulcer that is usually painful. It is frequently found in areas of trauma and may be mistaken clinically for a simple traumatic ulcer or even carcinoma. The causative organism is present in the base of these ulcers, making this a potential infectious hazard to dental personnel. Pharyngeal involvement results in painful ulcers and laryngeal lesions may cause dysphagia and voice changes.

Tuberculous gingivitis is an unusual form of tuberculosis which may appear as a diffuse, hyperemic, nodular, or papillary proliferation of the gingival tissues.

Tuberculosis may also involve the bone of the maxilla or mandible. One common mode of entry of organisms is an area of periapical inflammation by way of bloodstream, an anachoretic effect, or through the pulp chamber and root canal of a tooth with an open cavity. The lesion produced is essentially a tuberculous periapical granuloma or tuberculoma.

22.7 Tuberculous Osteomyelitis of Jaws

Tuberculous involvement of the mandible or maxilla is an occasional complication of pulmonary or disseminated tuberculosis. The organisms enter the bone by hematogenous route and set up a focus within the body of the mandible or maxilla (Figs. 22.1 and 22.2). The bone lesion is that of typical chronic osteomyelitis with a characteristic microscopic feature of tuberculous involvement. Tuberculous osteomyelitis frequently occurs in the later stages of the disease and has unfavorable prognosis.

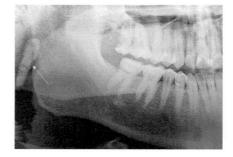

Fig. 22.1 A cropped panoramic view showing a chain radiopacity lateral to the ramus (yellow arrow). (Courtesy AZ. Syed, BDS, MHA, MS, Dipl. ABOMR)

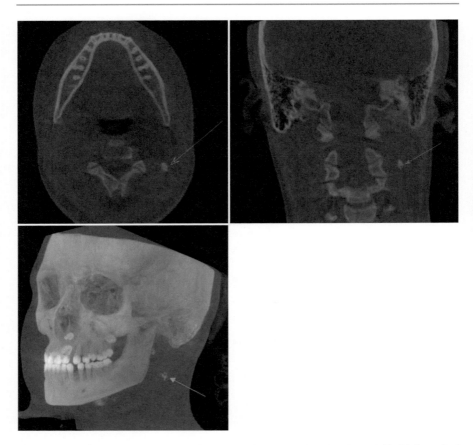

Fig. 22.2 CBCT axial and coronal sections and volume rendering showing calcified left cervical lymph node with matted appearance typical of tuberculous lymph node involvement. (Courtesy C. Matesi, DDS)

22.8 Scrofula

Drinking contaminated milk can result in a form of mycobacterial infection known as scrofula. Scrofula exhibits enlargement of the oropharyngeal lymphoid tissues and cervical lymph nodes. On occasion, the involved nodes may develop significant caseous necrosis and form numerous fistulas through the overlying skin.

22.9 Histopathology

The basic microscopic lesion of TB is granulomatous inflammation, in which granulomas show central caseous necrosis. In tissues *M. tuberculosis* incites a characteristic macrophage response in which focal zones of macrophages become surrounded by lymphocytes and fibroblasts. The macrophages develop an abundant eosinophilic cytoplasm, giving them a superficial resemblance to epithelial cells, in which case they are frequently called epithelioid cells.

Fusion of macrophages results in the appearance of Langhans giant cells, in which nuclei are distributed around the periphery of the cytoplasm. As the granulomas age, central necrosis occurs, which is usually referred to as caseous necrosis because of the gross cheesy texture of these zones.

The giant cells are notable in their appearance but are relatively few in number as compared with the mass of histiocytes in the zone of the tubercle. In the ulcer of the oral mucosa, the tubercle forms at or close to the oral epithelium, so that the stratified squamous epithelium undergoes necrosis and a large ulceration forms. The floor of the ulcer, as well as the walls, presents the characteristic pattern of a tubercle with necrosis, histiocytic and giant cell reaction, and lymphocytic infiltration. Because of the ulceration, polymorphonuclear leukocytes appear adjacent to the walls of the ulcer.

22.10 Diagnosis

The diagnosis of active infection must be confirmed by demonstration of the organisms by special microbial stains and culture of the infected tissue or sputum. The presence of acid-fast bacilli (AFB) in sputum smear is the gold standard for the diagnosis of TB. Imaging techniques like roentgenography of the affected part like chest and tuberculin test are most useful in supplementing the diagnosis of TB.

Identification of Mycobacteria from Respiratory Specimens: The demonstration of tubercle bacilli in a respiratory specimen like sputum is direct evidence of TB. WHO defines any patient whose sputum smear is positive for acid-fast bacilli as a case of pulmonary tuberculosis.

Mycobacterial Culture
Conventional mycobacterium culture is done on Lowenstein-Jensen medium; it takes 4–6 weeks for the growth of *M. tuberculosis*.

Tuberculin Test
The Mantoux test involves subcutaneous injection of 0.1 mL of 5 tuberculin units of purified protein derivative of Seibert stabilized with Tween 80 into the forearm. It is positive if induration is seen after 48–72 h. The maximum diameter of the induration is measured by palpation and interpreted as follows: more than 15 mm or ulceration strongly positive; more than 10 mm, positive; 5–9 mm, indeterminate; and <5 mm, negative. A positive reaction indicates that a mycobacterium has replicated in the tissues of the individual at some time but does not indicate an active disease.

Newer methods of diagnosis of TB include radioimmunoassay (RIA), soluble antigen fluorescent antibody (SAFA) test, enzyme-linked immunosorbent assay (ELISA), DNA probes, and polymerase chain reaction (PCR).

22.11 Treatment

Multiple drug therapy is often recommended as *M. tuberculosis* mutates and resists single drug therapy: isoniazid (INH) combined with rifampicin for 9 months or INH, rifampicin, and pyrazinamide for 2 months followed by INH and rifampicin for 4 months. Other drugs used are streptomycin and ethambutol.

Reference

1. Ananthanarayan r, jayaram pck. Textbook of microbiology. 4th ed. Orient longman, delhi. 1990.

Sarcoidosis

23

Contents

23.1	Etiology and Pathogenesis	109
23.2	Clinical Features	110
23.3	Oral Manifestations	111
23.4	Histopathologic Features	112
23.5	Treatment	113
References		113

Sarcoidosis is a multisystemic disorder of unknown cause that is characterized by the formation of immune granulomas in involved organs. Jonathan Hutchinson, an English surgeon-dermatologist, reported the first case of sarcoidosis in 1875. The term sarcoidosis was introduced later by Boeck in 1899, which in Greek means "flesh-like condition." Sarcoidosis affects all individuals regardless of race, sex, or age.

23.1 Etiology and Pathogenesis

Although the etiology of sarcoidosis is unknown, genetic, infectious, and environmental factors have been postulated as possible causes. A putative genetic pathogenesis has been suggested due to the presence of familial clusters in sarcoidosis. In addition, positive association with HLA-A1, HLA-B8, and HLA-DR3 has been identified. Studies confirm a genetic predisposition for sarcoidosis and present evidence for the allelic variation at the HLA-DRB1 locus as a major contributor. The genetic variations that promote susceptibility to the disease may reside in loci that influence the immune response.

© The Author(s), under exclusive license to Springer Nature Singapore Pte Ltd. 2024
K. Paiwal et al., *Handbook of Oral and Maxillofacial Giant Cell Lesions*,
https://doi.org/10.1007/978-981-97-2863-3_23

Infectious agents such as mycobacterium, propionibacteria, Epstein-Barr virus (EBV), and human herpesvirus-8 (HHV-8) have been considered as possible etiological agents, but so far, the scientific results have been inconsistent and inconclusive. Similarly, environmental factors (wood dust, pollen, clay, mold, silica) and occupational exposure (farmers, firefighters, military) have been suggested as etiological agents.

Reported evidence indicates an immunological response resulting from one or a combination of factors mentioned above. The T-helper 1 (Th1) lymphocytes play a central role in granuloma formation which is thought to be the result of deposition of poorly soluble antigenic material in the tissue. This antigenic material is taken up by antigen-presenting cells such as macrophages or dendritic cells, which then expose it to T lymphocytes. In response to these antigens, a local amplification of the cellular immune reaction takes place. In addition, mononuclear phagocytes and other inflammatory cells migrate to the site of the antigenic deposition under the influence of the chemokines and cytokines produced by Th1 cells. This results in the formation of a granuloma.

23.2 Clinical Features

Sarcoidosis is usually a self-limiting, benign disease with an insidious onset and protracted course. The disease exhibits a slight female predilection and a bimodal age distribution. The first peak is between the ages of 25 and 35 years and the second peak is at 45 and 65 years. Seasonal variations have been observed worldwide, with the peak incidence observed during late winter and early spring.

Sarcoidosis is a multi-organ disorder. The clinical symptoms depend on the ethnicity, chronicity of illness, site and extent of involvement of the organ, and activity of the granulomas. One third of the patients with sarcoidosis can present with nonspecific constitutional symptoms such as fever, fatigue and malaise, or weight loss. The most common presentation of sarcoidosis consists of pulmonary infiltration, hilar lymphadenopathy, and dermal and ocular lesions.

Although any organ may be affected, the lungs, lymph nodes, skin, eyes, and salivary glands are the predominant sites. Lymphoid tissue is involved in almost all cases. The mediastinal and paratracheal lymph nodes are involved commonly and chest radiographs frequently reveal bilateral hilar lymphadenopathy. Cutaneous manifestations occur about 25% of the time. These often appear as chronic, violaceous, indurated lesions that are termed **lupus pernio**. Lupus pernio is associated with poor prognosis of sarcoidosis and is associated with more severe pulmonary disease. Scattered, nonspecific, tender, erythematous nodules, known as erythema nodosum, frequently occur on the lower legs.

Sarcoidosis is a diagnosis of exclusion. No diagnostic tests or specific markers have been established yet. The diagnosis is based upon history (occupational or environmental exposure), pulmonary function tests (forced expiratory volume, vital capacity), hematology (complete blood count, erythrocyte sedimentation rate), biochemical investigations (liver and renal function tests, serum calcium and serum angiotensin-converting enzyme levels), chest radiograph, and histological studies.

Pulmonary function tests including forced expiratory volume, vital capacity, and diffusing capacity are all diminished. Hematological and biochemical tests may show anemia, lymphocytopenia, elevated ESR, increased liver enzymes, hypercalcemia, and hypercalcemic nephropathy. The serum angiotensin-converting enzyme (ACE) level is elevated in 50–80% of patients with sarcoidosis. It is useful in monitoring the disease progression and effectiveness of therapy. When serum ACE is used to diagnose sarcoidosis, it has a 10% false positive and a 40% false negative rate. The ACE level is also elevated in diabetes mellitus, cirrhosis, leprosy, and many other conditions. Therefore, ACE level has to be used as an adjunct, and a clinical correlation must be made for a specific diagnosis and disease progression or remission of sarcoidosis.

23.3 Oral Manifestations

Oral involvement in sarcoidosis is uncommon. Oral lesions are the first manifestation of the systemic sarcoidosis in the majority of the cases. Schroff [1] reported the first suspected case of sarcoid granulomas in the oral mucosa, but Poe [2] reported the first confirmed case of sarcoidosis affecting the oral cavity in the mandible.

The most frequently affected intraoral soft tissue site is the buccal mucosa, followed by the gingiva, lips, floor of the mouth, tongue, and palate. The common clinical presentations are localized swelling or nodules, ulcers, gingivitis, gingival hyperplasia, and gingival recession. The mucosal lesions may be normal in color, brownish-red, violaceous, or hyperkeratotic.

Intraosseous lesions affect either jaw and represent approximately one fourth of all reported intraoral cases (Fig. 23.1). Clinical manifestations when jaw bone is involved are mainly due to the lytic and permeative lesions in the bone. It includes loose teeth, pain radiating to the ears, nasal obstruction, and nonhealing socket.

The disease may also involve the salivary gland. The gland involvement is usually bilateral and is slightly more common in women. Submandibular and sublingual gland involvement is less common than parotid gland involvement. Clinical

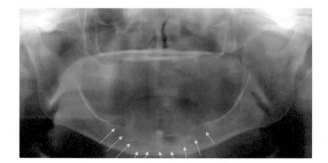

Fig. 23.1 Panoramic radiograph of a case of sarcoidosis involving and infiltrating the anterior mandibular region (yellow arrows)

presentation of sarcoidosis in major salivary glands is usually as painless firm swellings, and fluctuation in the size does not occur during the meal time. Xerostomia may also be present. Other rare but pathognomonic presentation of glandular involvement is Heerfordt syndrome. This syndrome is defined as systemic sarcoidosis characterized by parotitis (usually bilateral), uveitis, and facial nerve paralysis.

It is possible that some of the swellings seen on the mucosa of patients with sarcoidosis are actually expansions of localized involved minor salivary glands.

Differential Diagnosis
Depending on the lesion location:

1. Bony involvement alone can be mistaken for malignancy such as squamous cell carcinoma, leukemia, etc.
2. If nasopharynx is involved, it is difficult to differentiate from sinonasal lymphoma or sinonasal granulomatosis (Wegener's granulomatosis) on imaging

23.4 Histopathologic Features

Consistent microscopic findings of sarcoidosis are non-caseating granulomas. The center of the granulomas usually contains epithelioid macrophages surrounded by a rim of lymphocytes. Occasional multinucleated Langhans-type giant cells are also seen. The giant cells result from the fusion of the epithelioid mononuclear cells and may occasionally contain many inclusion bodies such as **Schumann bodies** or stellate asteroid bodies. Schumann bodies are basophilic, calcified, and laminated bodies derived from lysosomes found in about 48–88% of sarcoidosis patients. **Stellate or asteroid bodies** are found in 2–9% of the cases. They are spiculated in shape and represent entrapped collagen. Some lymph nodes may contain distinctive small yellow-brown bodies measuring 1–15 µm in the subcapsular sinus called **Hamazaki-Wesenberg bodies**. They represent large lysosomes and stain black with methenamine silver and red with periodic acid-Schiff stain. The histologic findings are not specific to sarcoidosis and may be found in other infectious granulomatous disorders.

Differential Diagnosis
The histologic differential diagnosis includes tuberculosis, Crohn's disease, leprosy, cat scratch disease, fungal infections (blastomycosis, coccidioidomycosis, and histoplasmosis), and parasitic diseases such as toxoplasmosis.

23.5 Treatment

Spontaneous resolution occurs in a significant number of patients. Corticosteroids are the drug of choice. Other agents may be used in addition or instead of corticosteroids. Chloroquine has been found to be useful in the management of this disease, either alone or in combination with corticosteroids. Immunosuppressive drugs are used in individuals not responding to corticosteroid management.

References

1. Schroff J. Sarcoid of the face (Besnier–Boeck–Schumann) disease: report of a case. JADA. 1942;29:2208–11.
2. Poe DL. Sarcoidosis of the jaw—A new disease of the mandible. Am J Orthod. 1943;29:52–6.

Herpes Simplex

24

(Acute Herpetic Gingivostomatitis, Herpes Labialis, Fever Blisters, Cold Sores)

Contents

24.1	Pathogenesis	116
24.2	Clinical Association of HSV-1 Infection	117
	24.2.1 Primary Herpetic Stomatitis	117
	24.2.2 Recurrent or Secondary Herpetic Labialis and Stomatitis	118
24.3	Clinical Features	118
24.4	Histological Features	119
24.5	Diagnosis	120
24.6	Treatment	120
References		120

Herpes simplex, an acute infectious disease, is probably the most common viral disease affecting man, with the exception of viral respiratory infections. HSV is a DNA virus and a member of the human herpesvirus (HHV) family, officially known as Herpetoviridae. Two types of HSVs are known to exist: type 1 (HSV-1 or HHV-1) and type 2 (HSV-2 or HHV-2).

Herpes simplex virus is composed of double-stranded DNA, protein capsid, tegument, and lipid envelope, which contains glycoproteins derived from the nuclear membrane of host cells. There are two immunologically different types of HSVs: type 1 and type 2. They differ antigenically and biologically but share 50% of the nucleotide sequence. Both are alphaviruses that are neurotropic and have a rapid replication cycle and broad host as well as cell range. These subtypes can be distinguished serologically or by restriction endonuclease analysis of the DNA.

The tissues preferentially involved by the herpes simplex virus (HSV), now often referred to as herpesvirus hominis, are derived from the ectoderm and consist principally of the skin, mucous membranes, eyes, and the central nervous system. A state of latency and reactivation is common in many viral infections, especially the herpes group. The incubation period is 1–26 days and can occur throughout the

© The Author(s), under exclusive license to Springer Nature Singapore Pte Ltd. 2024
K. Paiwal et al., *Handbook of Oral and Maxillofacial Giant Cell Lesions*,
https://doi.org/10.1007/978-981-97-2863-3_24

year. Transmission is mainly through close contact, kissing, sharing of glasses, cutlery or crockery, etc.

Gruter [1] was among the first to offer evidence that herpes simplex infection was caused by an infectious agent and that the fluid of vesicles from patients with herpes simplex would produce keratitis, when inoculated on sacrificed rabbit cornea.

Andrews [2] found that neutralizing antibodies against the herpes simplex virus were present in the circulating blood of most normal adults and persisted throughout life but that recurrent herpetic lesions frequently developed in these persons.

Dodd et al. [3] reported that the herpes simplex virus could be isolated from patients suffering from a gingivostomatitis with a particular clinical configuration.

These and other studies have finally led to the established principle that two types of infection with the herpes simplex virus occur. The first is a primary infection in a person who does not have circulating antibodies and the second is a recurrent infection in persons who have such antibodies. It is impossible to differentiate clinically between the lesions of a primary and a recurrent attack, although the primary infection is accompanied more frequently by severe systemic manifestations and is occasionally fatal. It has been shown, however, that most adults have circulating antibodies in the blood but have never exhibited a severe primary illness. Thus, it is reasoned, subclinical primary infections must be common.

There is an association between HSV-2 and carcinoma of the cervix. However, the link between HSV-1 and oral cancer is less compelling.

24.1 Pathogenesis

Mucosal surfaces and abraded skin favor the entry of virus and the initiation of replications in the cells of epidermis and dermis. The incubation period appears to range from 2 to 20 days, with an average of 6 days before development of lesions.

Initial or primary infection is asymptomatic and occurs commonly in childhood or infancy. Asymptomatic individuals periodically shed infectious HSV in saliva, observed in 2–9% of total cases. Viral shedding is usually greater in immunocompromised patients (approximately 38%) or in those undergoing oral surgery (approximately 20%). Asymptomatic shedding of HSV occurs principally during the prodrome phase of the primary disease.

Herpes simplex virus type 1 infects the oral mucosa by binding to specific cell surface receptors. In the host cell nucleus, the viral genome is replicated and structural proteins are synthesized and nucleocapsids assembled. Once inside the cell, replication results in the production of virions that ultimately cause cell death.

Following infection and local replication at mucosal surfaces, HSV-1 enters sensory nerve endings and is often transported by retrograde axonal transport to the neuronal cell bodies. Here, a more restricted replication cycle occurs, most often culminating in a latent infection of these neurons. Latency allows the maintenance of the viral genome in a nonpathogenic and non-replicate form and serves as a reservoir for later viral attack of the host. The trigeminal ganglion is the primary site of latency for HSV-1 and the lumbosacral ganglion for HSV-2, in which the virus remains present lifelong.

Though both subtypes produce orofacial and genital lesions, which are clinically indistinguishable, HSV-1 predominantly affects the face, lips, the oral cavity, and upper body skin, whereas HSV-2 usually affects the genitals and skin of the lower half of the body.

Once the primary infection resolves, the virus can no longer be recovered from ganglia but viral DNA can be found in the ganglion cells. Both humoral and cell-mediated immunity are responsible for the clinical manifestation, latency, and recurrence of the disease. Immunocompromised individuals, especially with impaired cellular immunity, are more prone for dissemination and recurrence or the primary disease.

24.2 Clinical Association of HSV-1 Infection

24.2.1 Primary Herpetic Stomatitis

Herpetic stomatitis is a common oral disease transmitted by droplet spread or contact with the lesions. It affects children and young adults.

It rarely occurs before the age of 6 months, apparently because of the presence of circulating antibodies in the infant derived from the mother. The disease occurring in children is frequently the primary attack and is characterized by the development of fever, irritability, headache, pain upon swallowing, and regional lymphadenopathy. Within a few days, the mouth becomes painful and the gingiva which is intensely inflamed appears erythematous and edematous. The lips, tongue, buccal mucosa, palate, pharynx, and tonsils may also be involved. Shortly thereafter yellowish, fluid-filled vesicles develop. These rupture and form shallow, ragged, extremely painful ulcers covered by a gray membrane and surrounded by an erythematous halo. The gingival inflammation precedes the formation of the ulcers by several days. The ulcers vary considerably in size, ranging from very tiny lesions to lesions measuring several millimeters or even a centimeter in diameter. They heal spontaneously within 7–14 days and leave no scar.

Utilizing culture techniques, August and Nordlund found that the HSV-1 could be isolated from facial, labial, and oral herpetic lesions for a mean duration of 3.5 days, with a range of 2–6 days, after the onset of the lesions, while HSV-2 could be isolated from genital lesions for a mean duration of 5.5 days, with a range of 2–14 days, after onset. Turner and his colleagues have shown that HSV could survive for 2–4 h on environmental surfaces such as cloth and plastic as well as on the skin of the hands contaminated by direct contact with labial or oral lesions.

HSV does not remain latent at the site of the original infection in the skin or oral mucosa. Instead, the virus reaches nerve ganglia supplying the affected areas, presumably along nerve pathways, and remains latent there until reactivated. Unfortunately, this incorporation of viral DNA into host DNA ensures a lifelong infection beyond the reach of antibody, cell-mediated immune responses, or chemotherapy.

24.2.2 Recurrent or Secondary Herpetic Labialis and Stomatitis

Recurrent herpetic stomatitis is usually seen in adult patients and manifests itself clinically as an attenuated form of the primary disease. It has been reported by Nahmias and Roizman that between 80% and 100% of adults in the lower socioeconomic levels have HSV-1 and/or HSV-2 circulating antibodies, whereas only 30–50% of adults in the higher socioeconomic levels, including medical, dental, and nursing personnel, have such antibodies. Those without antibodies are at higher risk of contact and infection, especially the latter groups because of the nature of their occupation.

The recurrent form of the disease is often associated with trauma, fatigue, menstruation, pregnancy, upper respiratory tract infection, emotional upset, allergy, exposure to sunlight or ultraviolet lamps, and gastrointestinal disturbances. The mechanism through which these various precipitating factors elicit an outbreak of lesions is unknown.

The viruses, once they have been introduced into the body, appear to reside dormantly within the regional ganglia. When reactivation is triggered, they spread along the nerves to sites on the oral mucosa and skin where they destroy the epithelial cells and induce the typical inflammatory response with the characteristic lesions of recurrent infection.

24.3 Clinical Features

Recurrent herpes simplex infection may occur at widely varying intervals, ranging from months to years. The lesions may develop either at the site of primary inoculation or in the adjacent area supplied by the involved ganglion. It may develop on the lips or intraorally. In either location, the lesions are frequently preceded by a burning or tingling sensation and a feeling of tautness, swelling, or slight soreness at the location in which the vesicles subsequently develop. These vesicles are generally small (1 mm or less in diameter), tend to occur in localized clusters, and may coalesce to form somewhat larger lesions. These gray or white vesicles rupture quickly, leaving a small red ulceration, sometimes with a slight erythematous halo. On the lips, these ruptured vesicles become covered by a brownish crust. The degree of pain present is quite variable.

It has been emphasized by Weathers and Griffin that the recurrent intraoral herpetic lesions almost invariably develop on oral mucosa that is tightly bound to the periosteum. Seldom do they occur on mobile mucosa, in contrast to the recurrent aphthous stomatitis which almost invariably occurs only on mobile mucosa. Thus,

24.4 Histological Features

The basic herpetic lesion is quite similar in both the primary and recurrent forms of the disease which differ only in their location and severity. Individual lesions involve the focal death of a group of cells within the spinous layer of the affected epithelium.

Liquefaction degeneration of these cells results in formation of an intraepithelial vesicle, whose central cavity is filled with a proteinaceous fluid. In the mucosa the vesicles tend to rupture early, but in the skin they may persist longer.

The abnormal cell division in epidermal cells creates multinucleated giant cells. So, these are the epidermal cells which are much larger than the normal and they contain multiple nuclei.

The infected cells are swollen and have pale eosinophilic cytoplasm and large vesicular nuclei, described as "ballooning degeneration." Balloon cells are frequently seen at the edge of the vesicle or may be found floating free in the fluid-filled cavity. They are degenerating epithelial cells that become swollen and round because of intracellular edema. When viewed by light microscopy, they appear to have lost their intracellular bridges due to acantholysis.

Cytoplasm of the infected cells forms giant cells. Multinucleated giant cells occasionally are found adjacent to the cavity of the vesicle and are seen more frequently in early lesions. The subjacent connective tissue is usually infiltrated by inflammatory cells.

Herpes simplex and herpes zoster viruses cause abnormal cell division in epidermal cells and this creates multinucleated giant cells. These are epidermal cells that are much larger than the normal epidermal cells. They contain multiple nuclei.

They are thought to result from the presence of the virus stimulating atypical nuclear proliferation without any equivalent division of cytoplasm in the infected cells. They were first noted by Tzanck and are sometimes referred as *Tzank cells*.

Intranuclear inclusion bodies present in the infected epithelial cells are the **Lipschutz bodies**. These are eosinophilic, ovoid, homogeneous structures within the nucleus, which tend to displace the nucleolus and nuclear chromatin peripherally. The displacement of chromatin often produces a peri-inclusion halo.

When the vesicle ruptures, the surface of the tissue is covered by exudate made up of fibrin, polymorphonuclear leukocytes, and degenerated cells. The lesions heal by peripheral epithelial proliferation.

24.5 Diagnosis

Herpes simplex can be diagnosed both clinically and by laboratory procedures. Scrapings obtained from the base of the lesions are stained with Wright's and Giemsa stains. PAP stain demonstrates balloon cells, multinucleated giant cells, and intranuclear inclusions.

Herpes simplex virus can be demonstrated in the laboratory by isolation of virus in tissue culture or by DNA in the scrapings from lesions. The most sensitive and accurate method for diagnosing these lesions is PCR technique.

24.6 Treatment

Antiviral drugs have a significant impact on the course of the disease, if it is diagnosed early. Antibiotic therapy helps in the prevention of secondary infection. Nonsteroidal anti-inflammatory drugs and topical anesthetic gel may relieve the discomfort considerably.

References

1. Gruter W. Experimentelle and Klinische Untersuchungen Uber Den Sog. Herpes Corneae Klin Monasbl Augenheilkd. 1920;65:398.
2. Andrews CH. Active immunisation in virus diseases. Br Med J. 1931;2:1036.
3. Dodd K, Johnston LM, Buddingh GJ. Herpetic stomatitis. J Pediatr. 1938;12:95.

Herpes Zoster

25

(Shingles, Zona)

Contents

25.1	Clinical Features	122
25.2	Oral Manifestations	122
25.3	Histological Features	123
25.4	Treatment	123

Herpes zoster is an acute infectious viral disease of an extremely painful and incapacitating nature which is characterized by inflammation of dorsal root ganglia or extramedullary cranial nerve ganglia, associated with vesicular eruptions of the skin or mucous membranes in areas supplied by the affected sensory nerves. The virus is the same as that of varicella or chicken pox (the VZ virus) and occasionally the two diseases are clinically nearly indistinguishable. It is now believed that herpes zoster is caused by reactivation of the latent VZ virus which had been acquired during a previous attack of chicken pox. In essence, a primary infection by the VZ virus results clinically in chicken pox, while a recurrent infection results clinically in herpes zoster.

Herpes zoster (shingles) is caused by reactivation of the varicella-zoster virus (VZV) from latency after infection with chicken pox. After acute infection, the virus lies dormant, typically for decades, in the sensory dorsal root ganglia. The cause for VZV reactivation is unclear. However, decline in cell-mediated immunity with age, certain diseases (such as HIV infection), or effects of immunosuppressive therapy are associated with reactivation of the virus.

Zoster occurs during the lifetime of 10–20% of individuals and the prevalence of attacks increases with age.

© The Author(s), under exclusive license to Springer Nature Singapore Pte Ltd. 2024
K. Paiwal et al., *Handbook of Oral and Maxillofacial Giant Cell Lesions*,
https://doi.org/10.1007/978-981-97-2863-3_25

25.1 Clinical Features

The disease is most common in adult life. It affects males and females with equal frequency. Although rare, it does occur in children.

Initially, the adult patient exhibits fever, general malaise, and pain and tenderness along the course of the involved sensory nerves, usually unilaterally. Often the nerve trunk is affected. Within a few days, the patient has a linear papular or vesicular eruption of the skin or mucosa supplied by the affected nerves. It is typically unilateral and dermatotic in distribution. After rupture of the vesicles, healing commences, although secondary infection may intervene and slow the process considerably.

25.2 Oral Manifestations

Herpes zoster may involve the face by infection of the trigeminal nerve. This usually consists of unilateral involvement of skin areas supplied by either the ophthalmic, maxillary, or mandibular nerves. The ophthalmic branch is affected several times more frequently than are the second or third divisions. This can lead to blindness secondary to corneal scarring. The involvement of maxillary and mandibular division causes facial and intraoral lesions.

Lesions of the oral mucosa are fairly common and extremely painful vesicles may be found on the buccal mucosa, tongue, uvula, pharynx, and larynx. These generally rupture to leave areas of erosion. One of the characteristic clinical features of the disease involving the face or oral cavity is the unilaterality of the lesions. Typically, when large, the lesions will extend up to the midline and stop abruptly.

A special form of zoster infection of the geniculate ganglion, with the involvement of the external ear and oral mucosa, has been termed Hunt's syndrome (James Ramsay Hunt's syndrome). The clinical manifestations include facial paralysis as well as pain of the external auditory meatus and pinna of the ear. In addition, vesicular eruptions occur in the oral cavity and oropharynx with hoarseness, tinnitus, vertigo, and occasional other disturbances.

When the neuralgia-associated pain persists longer than 3 months after the initial presentation of the acute rash, this is termed postherpetic neuralgia. This occurs in up to 15% of affected patients and at least 50% of patients older than 60 years of age. The pain is described as burning, throbbing, aching, itching, or stabbing, often with flares caused by light stroking of the area or from contact with adjacent clothing. Most of these neuralgias resolve within a year, with one half of the patient's experiencing resolution after 2 months.

25.3 Histological Features

Herpes zoster can frequently be recognized by the characteristic distribution of the lesions, although there may be a similarity to the lesions of herpes simplex infection. Skin lesions and oral lesions in particular may be easily identified as viral diseases by cytologic smears and the finding of characteristic multinucleated giant cells (Tzanck test) and intranuclear inclusions.

Infection by the herpes group of viruses can be rapidly and reliably diagnosed by a Tzanck test. Ideally, a vesicle <3 days old should be obtained since older lesions may get crusted or secondarily infected and the characteristic cytomorphology may no longer be present. The typical features include characteristic multinucleated syncytial giant cells and acantholytic cells. The cells appear as if they have been inflated (ballooning degeneration) and sometimes may grow tremendously, 60–80 μm in diameter.

The giant cells often have a tadpole, bipolar, or irregular teardrop shape with a smooth external contour, in sharp contrast to the jagged configuration of sheets of abraded normal squamous epithelium. Syncytial giant cells contain multiple nuclei (many with eight or more) that exhibit nuclear molding, so that the nuclei fit together in a jigsaw puzzle-like fashion. The nuclei show great variation in shape and size. Intranuclear inclusion bodies surrounded by subtle clear halo are characteristic of herpetic infection but are often difficult to find.

However, this does not differentiate between herpes zoster and herpes simplex. This can only be done by fluorescent antibody staining techniques, viral culture, or serologic diagnosis.

25.4 Treatment

Patients with herpes zoster and intact immune responses have generally been treated empirically. However, it has been shown that oral acyclovir used at high doses can shorten the disease course and reduce postherpetic pain. Analgesics provide only limited relief from pain. Topically applied substance P inhibitor (capsaicin) may provide relief from postherpetic pain. In patients with compromised immune responses, systemically administered acyclovir, vidarabine, or interferon is indicated.

Syphilis

26

Contents

26.1   Etiology.. 126
26.2   Mode of Transmission.. 126
26.3   Classification.. 127
      26.3.1   Stages of Acquired Syphilis.. 127
      26.3.2   Secondary Syphilis (Metastatic Syphilis)................................ 128
      26.3.3   Latent (Early and Late) Syphilis.. 128
      26.3.4   Congenital Syphilis.. 130
26.4   Histopathology... 130
26.5   Laboratory Diagnosis.. 131
      26.5.1   Direct Examination (Dark Field Examination)........................ 131
      26.5.2   Serologic Tests for Syphilis.. 131
26.6   Treatment and Prognosis... 132
References.. 132

Syphilis or lues is a chronic venereal infection caused by the spirochete *Treponema pallidum*. It is usually sexually transmitted and is characterized by episodes of active disease interrupted by periods of latency. The name "syphilis" was derived from a poem written by Fracastoro of Verona in 1530 describing the legend of a shepherd, the mythological handsome boy, Syphilus, who was cursed by Apollo with the disease. A complete history is summarized in Table 26.1.

In 1838 Philippe Ricord demonstrated conclusively that syphilis and gonorrhea were separate diseases on over 2500 human inoculations, and he was the first to propose a scheme for the categorization of syphilis into primary, secondary, and tertiary stages, which is still used today.

In 1905 Schaudinn and Hoffman demonstrated spirochetes in Giemsa-stained smears. August von Wassermann devised a serum reaction test for syphilis. The treatments for syphilis included mercury and organic arsenical compounds. In 1943 Mahoney successfully treated the first four cases with penicillin.

© The Author(s), under exclusive license to Springer Nature Singapore Pte
Ltd. 2024
K. Paiwal et al., *Handbook of Oral and Maxillofacial Giant Cell Lesions*,
https://doi.org/10.1007/978-981-97-2863-3_26

Table 26.1 Historical aspects of syphilis

Year	
1495	A widespread syphilis epidemic had spread through Europe [1]
1767	John Hunter considered that the diseases caused by *Neisseria gonorrhoeae* and *T. pallidum* were the same [2]
1838	Philippe Ricord: First to propose a scheme of syphilis into primary, secondary, and tertiary stages
1859	Bazin: Used the term lues maligna first time
1896	Third International Congress of Dermatology: Lues maligna was classified as the ulcerative form of secondary syphilis
1897	Neisser and Haslund: Classic description of lues maligna
1905	Schaudinn and Hoffman: demonstrated spirochetes in Giemsa-stained smears [3]
1906	Wassermann: developed the first serologic test for syphilis [4]
1943	Mahoney: first who successfully treated four cases of syphilis with penicillin [5]
1988	Shulkin: First to report HIV-infected patient with lues maligna

26.1 Etiology

Schaudinn and Hoffman [3] discovered the *Treponema pallidum* in syphilitic material. *Treponema pallidum* is one of the many spiral-shaped microorganisms which propel themselves by spinning around their longitudinal axis. *T. pallidum* is a thin, delicate filament 10 µm long that moves actively in fresh preparations. It is a fastidious spirochete whose only natural hosts are humans.

26.2 Mode of Transmission

Syphilitic infection can be transmitted by the following routes:

1. Sexual intercourse—common route of infection
2. Intimate person-to-person contacts with lesions on lips, tongue, or fingers
3. Transfusion of infected blood
4. Maternal–fetal transmission in congenital syphilis if the mother is infected

Sexual route of infection is the most common mode of contracting the infection. The organism is transmitted from such lesions during sexual intercourse across minute breaks in the skin or mucous membrane of the uninfected partner resulting in lesions on glans penis, vulva, vagina, and cervix, called as venereal syphilis. In recent years, there appears to have been an increase in the occurrence of extragenital syphilis as a result of an increase in orogenital activity and increased contact among infected male homosexuals; hence lesions may occur on the anus, lips, tongue, palate, gingiva, and breast.

26.3 Classification

Syphilis may be classified as either acquired or congenital, although this latter term is somewhat misleading, since the congenital form is "acquired" from an infected mother.

26.3.1 Stages of Acquired Syphilis

After acquiring the initial exposure to infection with *Treponema pallidum*, the spirochetes pass through the mucous membrane or skin and are then carried in the blood throughout the body. Once introduced into the body, the organisms are rapidly disseminated to the different sites by lymphatics and bloodstream. After an incubation period of about 3–6 weeks, an ulcerated lesion called a primary chancre develops at the site of entry, which is a painless, clean-based, indurated ulcer. The chancre starts as a papule but then superficial erosion occurs, resulting in the typical ulcer. The borders of the ulcers are raised, firm, and indurated. The base is usually smooth; the borders are raised and firm. The borders have a characteristic cartilaginous consistency. Occasionally secondary infections change the appearance, resulting in a painful lesion.

Most chancres are single, but multiple ulcers are sometimes seen particularly when skin folds are opposed to "kissing chancres." The primary chancre in males is usually on the penis, more specifically the coronal sulcus and glans. Anorectal chancres are common in homosexual men. In women, the commonest locations of the lesions, in order of decreasing frequency, are the labia majora, labia minora, fourchette, and perineum. The chancre resolves spontaneously over a period of 4–6 weeks to form a subtle scar. The chancre is usually associated with regional lymphadenopathy, which may be either unilateral or bilateral. The regional nodes are movable, discrete, and rubbery. Regional lymphadenopathy consisting of moderately enlarged, firm, nonsuppurative, painless lymph nodes usually accompanies the primary lesion. Spirochetes are readily demonstrable in the material scraped from the base of the ulcer, using dark field microscopy.

Oral Manifestations
About 95% of the chancres occur on the genitalia but extragenital primary lesions occur in about 4.5–12% of the patients with syphilis. This extragenital syphilis is a result of an increase in orogenital activity and increased contact among infected male homosexuals. A chancre of the lip is the most common extragenital lesion accounting for about 60% of cases and may present at the angles of the mouth. Other sites affected are the tongue, palate, gingiva, and tonsils. Intraoral chancres are usually slightly painful due to secondary bacterial infection.

The lesions are infectious, and other modes of transmission are through kissing and intermediate contact with cups, glasses, eating utensils, and medical as well as dental instruments.

26.3.2 Secondary Syphilis (Metastatic Syphilis)

This stage usually commences about 6 weeks after the primary lesion. It is characterized by diffuse eruptions of the skin and mucous membranes. During secondary syphilis, systemic symptoms often arise. The most common are painless lymphadenopathy, sore throat, malaise, headache, weight loss, fever, and musculoskeletal pain. The signs of secondary syphilis are variable: generalized skin lesions in 75%, mucosal ulcers in 33%, and generalized lymphadenopathy in 50% of cases. The skin lesions are found predominantly on the face, hands, feet, and genitalia. The skin lesions appear as dull red macular or papular spots.

Occasionally, papillary lesions that resemble viral papillomas may arise during this time and are known as condylomata lata. Sometimes, especially in the presence of a compromised immune system, secondary syphilis can exhibit an explosive and widespread form known as lues maligna. This term has prodromal symptoms of fever, headache, and myalgia, followed by the formation of necrotic ulcerations, which commonly involve the face and scalp. In contrast to the isolated chancre noted in the primary stage, multiple lesions are typical of secondary syphilis.

Oral Manifestations

They are classically slightly raised, greenish-white, glistening patches on the mucous membrane of the tonsils, soft palate, tongue, or cheek but rarely the gingival tissues. The "mucous patches" are usually multiple, painless, grayish-white plaques overlying an ulcerated surface, commonly occurring on the tongue or gingival or buccal mucosa, and are highly infectious. Lesions which form on the larynx and pharynx may lead to hoarseness. Mucous patches coalesce to produce a serpiginous lesion called a "snail-track ulcer." Cervical lymph nodes enlarge and become rubbery in consistency. In recent years the secondary syphilitic lesions found in the mouth are atypical, due to inadequate treatment as a result of antibiotic therapy for an unrelated infection. The secondary stage lesions may undergo spontaneous remission within a few weeks, but exacerbations may continue to occur for months or several years.

26.3.3 Latent (Early and Late) Syphilis

Latent syphilis is a stage in which patients are seroreactive but asymptomatic. It occurs between the disappearance of secondary syphilis symptoms and the appearance of tertiary syphilis manifestations or therapeutic cure. About 90% of first relapses occur within 1 year, it is defined as early latent syphilis, and late latent syphilis is defined as occurring after 1 year.

Tertiary Syphilis

Tertiary syphilis develops in approximately one third of the untreated patients, usually after a latent period of 5 years or more. This period of latency may last from 1 to 30 years. Latency has been divided into two stages:

1. Early latency

   It encompasses the first year after infection.
2. Late latency

   Late latent syphilis beginning 1 year after infection in the untreated patient is associated with relative immunity to infectious relapse and with increasing resistance to reinfection. Pregnant women with latent syphilis may infect the fetus in utero.

The third stage, which is known as tertiary syphilis, develops after the latency period. The characteristic lesion is the gumma. They typically develop from 1 to 10 years after the initial infection and may involve any part of the body. Although they may be very destructive, they respond rapidly to treatment and therefore are relatively benign. Gummas may be solitary or multiple. They are usually asymmetric and are often grouped. They may start as a superficial nodule or as a deeper lesion that breaks down to form punched-out ulcers. They are indurated on palpation. There, often, is central healing with an atrophic scar surrounded by hyperpigmented borders.

Gummas develop in the skin, the mucous membranes, and bones. The other organs involved in tertiary syphilis are the cardiovascular and the nervous system. In the cardiovascular system, there will be aneurysm of the ascending aorta and left ventricular hypertrophy, and congestive heart failure may occur. Involvement of the central nervous system may result in tabes dorsalis, psychosis, dementia, paresis, and death.

Oral Manifestations

The intraoral gumma most commonly involves the tongue and palate, although the soft palate, the lips, and face are also relatively commonly involved. In case of palate, the gumma may eventually perforate into the nasal cavity by sloughing off the necrotic mass of tissue. The palatal lesions are usually midline.

Syphilitic osteomyelitis, involving the mandible and less commonly the maxillae, has occasionally been described. The condition is characterized by pain, swelling, suppuration, and sequestration and both clinically and radiographically, the condition may resemble pyogenic osteomyelitis. If ossification occurs in the lesion, the radiographic appearance of the affected area may be similar to that of an osteogenic sarcoma.

Atrophic or interstitial glossitis (luetic glossitis) is another oral manifestation of tertiary syphilis. Clinically, there is atrophy of the filiform and fungiform papillae, which results in a smooth, sometimes wrinkled lingual surface. In the past, this form of atrophic glossitis was thought to be precancerous. Syphilis very rarely affects the salivary glands but both secondary and tertiary lesions have been described in the parotid glands.

26.3.4 Congenital Syphilis

Congenital or prenatal syphilis is transmitted to the offspring only by an infected mother and is not inherited. Sir Jonathan Hutchinson (1858) described changes found in congenital syphilis and defined the following three pathognomonic diagnostic features, known as "Hutchinson's triad."

1. Hutchinson's teeth
2. Ocular interstitial keratitis
3. Eighth nerve deafness

The infection alters the formation of both the anterior teeth (Hutchinson's incisors) and the posterior dentition (mulberry molars, Fournier's molars, Moon's molars). Hutchinson's incisors resemble a straight edge screwdriver often exhibiting a central hypoplastic notch. Mulberry molars taper toward the occlusal surface, with a constructed grinding surface and abnormal occlusal anatomy with numerous disorganized globular projections that resemble the surface of a mulberry.

Interstitial keratitis of the eyes is not present at birth but usually develops between the ages of 5 and 25 years. The affected eye has a pacified corneal surface with a resultant loss of visions.

Other features of congenital syphilis are as follows: frontal bossing, short maxilla, high-arched palate, saddle nose, Higoumenakis sign or irregular thickening of the sternoclavicular portion of the clavicle, relative prognathism of the mandible, rhagades, saber shins, and scaphoid scapula.

26.4 Histopathology

Chancre appears as a superficial ulcer characterized by dense infiltrate of lymphocytes, plasma cells, and few macrophages. Perivascular aggregation of mononuclear cells particularly plasma cells (periarteritis and endarteritis) is also observed. The microorganisms present in the lesion may be demonstrable by silver staining.

Mucocutaneous lesions during secondary syphilis reveal the characteristic proliferative endarteritis, accompanied by lymphoplasmocytic inflammatory infiltrate. Spirochetes can be easily demonstrated.

Microscopically the gumma is a granuloma. It shows central coagulative necrosis resembling caseation but is less destructive so that outlines of necrosed cells can still be faintly seen with surrounding zone of palisaded macrophages along with lymphocytes, plasma cells, giant cells, and fibroblasts.

26.5 Laboratory Diagnosis

26.5.1 Direct Examination (Dark Field Examination)

The serum exudate is collected by applying gentle pressure at the base of the lesion, and wet films are prepared after applying a thin coverslip, examined under dark field microscopy. *T. pallidum* is identified by its slender spiral structure and slow movement. This technique has a limited value in the lesions of the mouth since the oral commensal *T. microdentium* closely resembles *T. pallidum*.

However, specific immunofluorescence tests, such as direct fluorescent antibody test for *T. pallidum* (DFA-TP), are helpful in diagnosis. This test is done using fluorescent tagged anti-*T. pallidum* antiserum.

26.5.2 Serologic Tests for Syphilis

Tests for syphilis can be classified as follows:

1. Nonspecific Tests
   (a) Anticardiolipin antibodies; standard test for syphilis; STS

   Wassermann complement reaction test: uses purified lipid extract of beef heart called lipoprotein, with added lecithin and cholesterol. This test is no longer used and is replaced by a simpler flocculation test.

   Flocculation test of Khan was the first flocculation test used and is now replaced by the more rapid VDRL tests.
   (b) VDRL (Venereal Disease Research Laboratories) test (slide flocculation)

   The inactivated serum (heated at 56° for 3 min) is mixed with cardiolipin antigen on a special slide and rotated for 4 min. Cardiolipin remains as uniform crystals in the normal serum but forms visible clumps on combining with the regained antibody. The reaction is read under a low-power microscope.

   Modifications: Rapid plasma reagin (RPR) test uses VDRL antigen containing fine carbon particles, which make the results evident to the naked eyes.
2. Specific Treponemal Antibodies
   (a) *Treponema pallidum* immobilization (TPI) test: The test serum is incubated with the complement as well as *T. pallidum* and maintained in a complex medium anaerobically. If antibodies are present, the treponemes will be immobilized when observed under dark field illumination.

   Results:
   - Positive—if the percentage of treponemes immobilized is 50 or more
   - Negative—if the percentage of treponemes immobilized is 20
   - Inconclusive—if treponemes are 20–50%

(b) FTA-ABS (fluorescent treponemal antibody absorption) test
   The test serum is preabsorbed with a sonicate of Reiter treponemes. This is a confirmatory and diagnostic test, not for routine screening.
(c) MHA-TP (microhemagglutination assay for *Treponema pallidum*) is similar to FTA-ABS but can be qualified and automated.

These tests become positive from the time of development of the first lesion which remain positive for life and therefore are not useful in diagnosis of second incidence of infection. Therefore, organisms should be demonstrated in case of reinfection within the tissues or exudates. The laboratory diagnosis of syphilis is usually made by serology since *T. pallidum* cannot be routinely cultured in vitro.

26.6 Treatment and Prognosis

The treatment for syphilis necessitates an individual evaluation and a customized therapeutic approach. The treatment of choice is penicillin. Erythromycin or tetracycline is given to patients who are allergic to penicillin.

References

1. https://pubmed.ncbi.nlm.nih.gov/15252975/.
2. https://link.springer.com/chapter/10.1007/978-1-4471-2068-1_4.
3. Schaudinn FN, Hoffman E. Vorlaufiger Bericht Uber Das Vorkommen von Spirochaeten in Syphilitischen Krankheits Produkten Und Bei Papillomen. Arbeiten K Gesundheits. 1905;22:527–34.
4. Wassermann A, Neisser A, Bruck C. Eine Serodiagnostische Reaktion Bei Syphilis. Dtsch Med Wochenschr. 1906;32:745–6.
5. Mahoney JF, Arnold RC, Harris AD. Penicillin treatment of early syphilis. Am J Public Health. 1943;33:1387–91.

Leprosy

(Hansen's Disease)

27

Contents

27.1	Pathogenesis	133
27.2	Clinical Features	134
27.3	Oral Manifestations	134
27.4	Histopathologic Features	135
27.5	Treatment	135

Leprosy is a chronic infectious granulomatous disease caused by *Mycobacterium leprae* (*M. leprae*). It affects mainly the skin and peripheral nerves. It may also affect internal organs and mucosa.

27.1 Pathogenesis

An immunologic and epidemiological study suggests most people develop a subclinical infection and very few develop infection. Once infected, both cell-mediated and humoral responses are elicited by bacterial antigen DNA glycolipids. Lipoarabinomannan, a component of the cell membrane, induces immune suppression by inhibiting the interferon gamma-mediated activation of macrophages.

The bacteria are taken by histiocytes in the skin and Schwann cells in the nerves. This usually results in an inflammatory response involving histiocytes and lymphocytes. It is clinically called an indeterminate type represented as a hypopigmented or erythematous macule. The clinical spectrum and ultimate outcome of disease depend upon the intensity of specific cell-mediated immunity. Individuals prone to tuberculoid type have an intense cell-mediated immune response and low bacillary load, whereas patients with lepromatous type have low specific cell-mediated immune response and a high bacillary load. These two different types are genetically controlled.

© The Author(s), under exclusive license to Springer Nature Singapore Pte Ltd. 2024
K. Paiwal et al., *Handbook of Oral and Maxillofacial Giant Cell Lesions*,
https://doi.org/10.1007/978-981-97-2863-3_27

27.2 Clinical Features

Leprosy manifests in two polar forms, namely, tuberculoid type and lepromatous type. Between these two the borderline and indeterminate forms occur, depending upon the host response.

Currently, leprosy is classified into two separate categories, paucibacillary and multibacillary. Paucibacillary leprosy corresponds closely to the tuberculoid pattern of leprosy and exhibits a small number of well-circumscribed, hypopigmented skin lesions. Nerve involvement usually results in anesthesia of the affected skin, often accompanied by a loss of sweating. Oral lesions are rare in this variant.

Multibacillary leprosy corresponds well to the lepromatous pattern of leprosy and begins slowly with numerous, ill-defined, hypopigmented macules or papules on the skin that, with time, become thickened. The face is a common site of involvement and the skin enlargements can lead to a distorted facial appearance (*leonine facies*). Hairs, including the eyebrows and lashes, are often lost. Nerve involvement leads to loss of sweating and decreased light touch, pain, as well as temperature sensors. This sensory loss begins in the extremities and spreads to most of the body. Nasal involvement results in nosebleeds, stuffiness, and a loss of the sense of smell. The hard tissue of the floor, septum, and bridge of the nose may be affected. Collapse of the bridge of the nose is considered pathognomonic.

27.3 Oral Manifestations

Oral lesions are uncommon in leprosy but when present occur in patients with the lepromatous form. These lesions are generally asymptomatic ulcers or nodules sometimes rich in *M. leprae* resembling nonspecific oral lesions.

The locations affected in order of frequency are the hard palate, soft palate, labial maxillary gingiva, tongue, lips, buccal maxillary gingiva, labial mandibular gingiva, and buccal mucosa. Affected soft tissue initially appears as yellowish to red, sessile, firm, enlarging papules that develop ulceration and necrosis, followed by attempted healing by secondary intention. Continuous infection of an area can led to significant scarring and loss of tissue. Complete loss of the uvula and fixation of the soft palate may occur. The lingual lesions appear primarily in the anterior third and often begin as areas of erosion, which may develop into large nodules. Infection of the lip can result in significant macrocheilia.

Direct infiltration of the inflammatory process associated with lepromatous leprosy can destroy the bone underlying the areas of soft tissue involvement. Often the infection creates a unique pattern of facial destruction that has been termed *facies leprosa* and demonstrates a triad of lesions consisting of atrophy of the anterior nasal spine, atrophy of the anterior maxillary alveolar ridge, and endonasal inflammatory changes.

Involvement of the anterior maxilla can result in significant bone erosion, with loss of the teeth in this area. Maxillary involvement in children can affect the developing teeth which will produce enamel hypoplasia and short tapering roots. The facial and trigeminal nerves can also be involved with the infectious process.

27.4 Histopathologic Features

Biopsy specimens of paucibacillary leprosy typically reveal the tuberculoid pattern that demonstrates granulomatous inflammation with well-formed clusters of epithelioid histiocytes, lymphocytes, and multinucleated giant cells. There is a paucity of organisms; when present, they can be demonstrated only when stained with acid-fast stains, such as the Fite method.

Multibacillary leprosy is associated with a lepromatous pattern that demonstrates no well-formed granulomas; the typical finding is sheets of lymphocytes intermixed with vacuolated histiocytes known as lepra cells. Unlike tuberculoid leprosy, an abundance of organisms can be demonstrated with acid-fast stains in the lepromatous variant.

27.5 Treatment

Specific long-term chemotherapy is initiated upon diagnosis. Rifampicin and dapsone for 6 months in case of tuberculoid type and rifampicin and dapsone along with clofazimine in case of lepromatous type are usually advocated.

Osteomyelitis

28

Contents

28.1 Acute Osteomyelitis.. 137
    28.1.1 Histological Features.. 138
28.2 Chronic Osteomyelitis.. 138
    28.2.1 Histological Features.. 138
28.3 Radiographic Features.. 138
28.4 Differential Diagnosis.. 140
28.5 Treatment.. 140

Osteomyelitis is usually defined as the inflammation of the bone and its marrow contents. Changes in the calcified tissue are secondary to inflammation of the soft tissue component of the bone. The term osteomyelitis is reserved for infections which spread through the bone to a larger extent. Though osteomyelitis commonly occurs as a complication of dental sepsis, it is also seen in various other situations.

Predisposing factors include fractures due to trauma and road traffic accidents, gunshot wounds, radiation damage, Paget's disease, and osteoporosis. Systemic conditions like malnutrition, acute leukemia, uncontrolled diabetes mellitus, sickle cell anemia, and chronic alcoholism may also predispose to osteomyelitis. The disease may be acute, subacute, or chronic and presents different clinical course, depending upon its nature.

28.1 Acute Osteomyelitis

Acute suppurative osteomyelitis of the jaw is a serious sequela of periapical infection. The patient has severe pain, trismus, and paresthesia of the lips in case of mandibular involvement and manifests an elevation of temperature with regional

© The Author(s), under exclusive license to Springer Nature Singapore Pte Ltd. 2024
K. Paiwal et al., *Handbook of Oral and Maxillofacial Giant Cell Lesions*, https://doi.org/10.1007/978-981-97-2863-3_28

lymphadenopathy. The white blood cell count is frequently elevated. The teeth in the area of involvement are loose and sore. Pus may exude from the gingival margin.

28.1.1 Histological Features

The medullary spaces are filled with exudates. The inflammatory cells are chiefly neutrophils with occasional lymphocytes and plasma cells. The osteoblasts bordering the bony trabeculae are generally destroyed. Bony trabeculae show reduced osteoblastic activity and increased osteoclastic resorption.

28.2 Chronic Osteomyelitis

Chronic osteomyelitis may be one of the sequelae of acute osteomyelitis or it may represent a long-term, low-grade inflammatory reaction. The mandible is affected more commonly than the maxilla. Pain is usually present but varies in intensity. Swelling of the jaw is commonly encountered; loose teeth and sinus tracts are seen less often.

28.2.1 Histological Features

The inflammatory reaction in chronic osteomyelitis varies from very mild to intense. A few chronic inflammatory cells (lymphocyte and plasma cells) are seen in fibrous marrow. Both osteoblastic and osteoclastic activity may be seen, along with irregular bony trabeculae. In advanced cases, necrotic bone (sequestrum) may be present. Reversal lines reflect the waves of deposition and resorption of bone. Inflammatory cells are more numerous and osteoclastic activity is more prominent in advanced cases with respect to milder ones.

28.3 Radiographic Features

The imaging features of this condition might vary based on the stage of the disease. In the acute and early phase, even though inflammatory changes and symptoms are observed in clinical and histological level, it might not be evident radiographically until around 30–40% of demineralization occurs. In the acute phase, the margins are ill-defined and the trabeculae decrease in density. As the entity takes a chronic course, the margins become more defined and have a wide zone of transition. Areas of radiolucency appear scattered and as time progresses, sclerotic areas appear within the lytic areas (Fig. 28.1). Apparently, as the sclerosis becomes denser, the nonviable bone gets separated from the underlying bone forming sequestrum. The sequestrum appears radiographically as a dense radiopaque entity surrounded by a

28.3 Radiographic Features

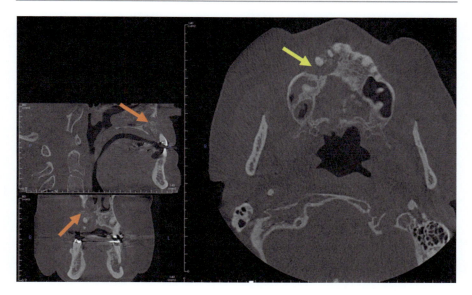

Fig. 28.1 Axial, sagittal, and coronal sections of CBCT of a case of osteomyelitis showing diffuse predominantly radiolucent lesion in the right maxilla (yellow arrows) with radiopaque areas (sequestra) within the entity (orange arrow). The labial cortical plate is lost. (Courtesy AZ. Syed, BDS, MHA, MS, Dipl. ABOMR)

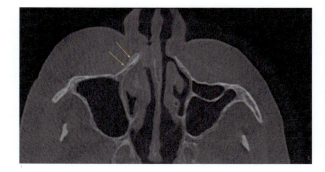

Fig. 28.2 CBCT axial section of chronic osteomyelitis showing periosteal reaction on the anterior surface of the right maxilla (yellow arrows)

zone of radiolucency (Fig. 28.2). The inflammatory exudate may accumulate under the periosteum, lifting it from the bone surface, thus stimulating new bone formation. This periosteal reaction creates an "onion peel" appearance where one or more alternating radiopaque and radiolucent lines run parallel to the bone surface. With progression, bone deposition obliterates the radiolucent areas and creates a uniform radiopacity. This condition is called proliferative periostitis, most commonly seen in children. In some cases, fistula formation occurs with a break in the cortex. Lamina dura of the involved teeth becomes less apparent along with widening of the periodontal ligament space.

28.4 Differential Diagnosis

1. **Squamous Cell Carcinoma:** Destructive bony lesion without periosteal reaction and sequestrum. Clinical examination may reveal soft tissue mass and fixed non-movable lymph nodes.
2. **Medication-Related Osteonecrosis/Osteoradionecrosis:** Clinical history of exposed bone, medication history, or prior radiation therapy helps in differentiating. Low propensity for periosteal reaction.
3. **Fibrous Dysplasia:** Expanded cortex is intact without periosteal bone reaction or bony sequestration or clinical signs of infection.
4. **Osteosarcoma:** More destructive behavior. Periosteal bone reaction has a sunray pattern and clinically may be associated with a rapid growing mass.
5. **Metastasis:** Clinical history of primary tumor and no source of infection.

28.5 Treatment

The basic treatment of osteomyelitis centers around the selection of appropriate antibiotics and proper timing of surgical intervention.

Measles

29

(Rubeola)

Contents

29.1	Epidemiology	141
29.2	Clinical Features	142
29.3	Oral Manifestations	142
29.4	Histopathologic Features	143
29.5	Treatment	143

Measles is an ancient disease, but for a long time, no distinction was made between measles and other exanthematous diseases, including smallpox. It was only in 1629 that measles came to be considered as a separate entity. Thomas Sydenham in 1690 gave the first clear and accurate description of measles in the English language.

Measles is an acute, contagious, dermotropic viral infection, primarily affecting children and occurring many times in epidemic form. It is caused by paramyxovirus belonging to the family Paramyxoviridae, which is an RNA virus. Outbreaks are often cyclic in their appearance and are seen commonly at 2- or 3-year intervals. Spread of the disease occurs by direct contact with an affected person or by droplet infection; the portal of entry is the respiratory tract.

29.1 Epidemiology

Measles is endemic throughout the world and produces epidemics every 2–3 years. Epidemics are usually seen in late winter and early spring, with a peak in April. The disease has maximum incidence in children 1–5 years of age. It is uncommon in the first 6 months of life due to the presence of maternal antibodies. One attack confers solid immunity. Man is the only natural host for measles.

© The Author(s), under exclusive license to Springer Nature Singapore Pte Ltd. 2024
K. Paiwal et al., *Handbook of Oral and Maxillofacial Giant Cell Lesions*, https://doi.org/10.1007/978-981-97-2863-3_29

Measles is contagious from the first or second day even before the onset of serious illness or appearance of rash. It is transmitted mainly through respiratory secretions and also through direct contact of droplets. The incubation period is generally from 8 to 12 days. It is mainly transmitted in large families, crowded homes, and slums. It is a self-limiting disease in healthy immunocompetent children, but morbidity and mortality are high in malnourished and immunocompromised individuals.

29.2 Clinical Features

The disease has an incubation period of 10–12 days and begins with prodromal symptoms of fever, malaise, coryza (running nose), conjunctivitis, and cough. The exanthematous rash follows after a few days and lasts from 4 to 7 days. The face is involved first, with eventual downward spread to the trunk and extremities. Ultimately, a diffuse erythematous maculopapular eruption is formed. The rash clears in a similar downward progression and is replaced by a brown pigmentary staining.

Common complications in young children are otitis pneumonia, persistent bronchitis, and diarrhea, the less common complication being encephalitis and a delayed complication termed subacute sclerosing panencephalitis (SSPE) which can arise as late as 11 years after the initial infection. It can lead to personality changes, seizures, coma, and death. Measles in immunocompromised patients can be serious, with a high risk of complications and death.

29.3 Oral Manifestations

The oral lesions are prodromal, frequently occurring 2–3 days before the cutaneous rash, and are pathognomonic of this disease. These intraoral lesions are called **Koplik's spots**.

Henry Koplik, a New York pediatrician, described these highly characteristic and pathognomonic lesions in 1896. They are tiny 1–2 mm white spots, often with a red rim. These little necrotic areas are usually opposite the molars or grouped around the parotid duct opening. The number of Koplik's spots may range from a few to more than 100.

They are reported to occur in as high as 97% of all patients with measles. Immune reaction to the virus in the endothelial cells of dermal capillaries plays a role in the development of spots. The spots disappear after the onset of rash. These spots usually appear on the buccal mucosa and are small and irregularly shaped flecks which appear as bluish-white specks surrounded by a bright-red margin. These macular lesions increase in number rapidly and coalesce to form small patches. Palatal and pharyngeal petechiae, generalized inflammation, congestion, swelling, and focal ulceration of the gingiva, palate, as well as throat may also occur.

29.4 Histopathologic Features

Initially, Koplik's spots represent areas of focal hyperparakeratosis in which the underlying epithelium exhibits spongiosis, intercellular edema, dyskeratosis, and epithelial syncytial giant cells. The number of nuclei within these giant cells ranges from 3 to over 25. Close examination of the epithelial cells often reveals pink-staining inclusions in the nuclei or less commonly in the cytoplasm. Upon electron microscopy, the inclusions have been shown to represent microtubular aggregates characteristic of the causative paramyxovirus. As the spot ages, the epithelium exhibits heavy exocytosis by neutrophils leading to microabscess formation, epithelial necrosis, and ultimately ulceration.

Examination of hyperplastic lymphoid tissue during the prodromal stage of measles reveals a similar alteration. Within the hyperplastic lymphoid tissue, there are numerous multinucleated giant lymphocytes. These multinucleated cells subsequently have been termed **Warthin-Finkeldey giant cells** and were thought for a time to be specific for measles. Since that time, however, similar appearing cells have been noted in a variety of lymphoproliferative disorders such as lymphoma, Kimura's disease, AIDS-related lymphoproliferative disease, and lupus erythematosus.

29.5 Treatment

There is no specific treatment for measles. Supportive therapy of bed rest, fluids, adequate diet, and analgesics generally suffices.

Histoplasmosis

30

Contents

30.1	Clinical Features	145
30.2	Oral Manifestations	146
30.3	Histological Features	146
30.4	Treatment	146

Histoplasmosis is a generalized fungus infection caused by the organism *Histoplasma capsulatum*. *H. capsulatum* is dimorphic, growing as yeast at body temperature in the human host and as a mold in its natural environment. It is usually acquired by inhalation of dust containing spores of the fungus, the contamination probably occurring from excreta of birds.

30.1 Clinical Features

The disease is characterized by a chronic low-grade fever, productive cough, splenomegaly, hepatomegaly, and lymphadenopathy, since the organisms have a special predilection for the reticuloendothelial system and chiefly involve the spleen, liver, lymph nodes, and bone marrow. Anemia and leukopenia also may be present. The infection by this organism may be extremely mild, manifesting only local lesions such as subcutaneous nodules or suppurative arthritis. Histoplasmosis often terminated fatally, particularly the generalized form.

© The Author(s), under exclusive license to Springer Nature Singapore Pte Ltd. 2024
K. Paiwal et al., *Handbook of Oral and Maxillofacial Giant Cell Lesions*,
https://doi.org/10.1007/978-981-97-2863-3_30

30.2 Oral Manifestations

They appear as nodular, ulcerative, or vegetative lesions on the buccal mucosa, gingiva, tongue, palate, or lips. The ulcerated areas are usually covered by a nonspecific gray membrane and are indurated.

30.3 Histological Features

Histoplasmosis appears basically to be a granulomatous infection which affects chiefly the reticuloendothelial system. Microscopic examination of lesional tissue shows either a diffuse infiltrate of macrophages or more commonly collection of macrophages organized into granulomas. Multinucleated giant cells are usually seen in association with the granulomatous inflammation.

The causative organism can be identified with some difficulty in the routine hematoxylin and eosin-stained section. Special stains, such as the PAS and Grocott-Gomori methenamine silver, readily demonstrate the characteristics of *H. capsulatum*.

30.4 Treatment

Acute histoplasmosis is a self-limiting process and requires no specific treatment. Chronic histoplasmosis is usually treated by intravenous amphotericin B.

Cryptococcosis

31

(Torulosis, European Blastomycosis)

Contents

31.1	Clinical Features	147
31.2	Oral Manifestations	148
31.3	Histological Features	148
31.4	Treatment and Prognosis	148

Cryptococcosis is a relatively uncommon fungal disease caused by the yeast *Cryptococcus neoformans*. This organism normally causes no problem in immunocompetent people, but it can be devastating to the immunocompromised patient.

The disease is acquired by inhalation of *C. neoformans* spores into the lungs, resulting in an immediate influx of neutrophils that destroy most of the yeasts. Macrophages soon follow, although resolution of infection in the immunocompetent host ultimately depends on an intact cell-mediated immune system.

31.1 Clinical Features

Primary cryptococcal infection of the lungs is often asymptomatic; however, a mild flu-like illness may develop. Patients complain of productive cough, chest pain, fever, and malaise. Dissemination of the infection is common in immunocompromised patients, and the most frequent site of involvement is the meninges, followed by the skin, bone, and prostate gland.

Cryptococcal meningitis is characterized by headache, fever, vomiting, and neck stiffness. In many instances, this is the initial sign of the disease. Cutaneous lesions develop in 10–20% of patients with disseminated disease. The skin of the head and neck is often involved. The lesions appear as erythematous papules or pustules that may ulcerate, discharging pus-like material rich in cryptococcal organisms.

© The Author(s), under exclusive license to Springer Nature Singapore Pte Ltd. 2024
K. Paiwal et al., *Handbook of Oral and Maxillofacial Giant Cell Lesions*,
https://doi.org/10.1007/978-981-97-2863-3_31

31.2 Oral Manifestations

Although oral lesions are relatively rare, they have been described as craterlike, nonhealing ulcers that are tender on palpation. Dissemination to salivary gland tissue also has been reported rarely.

31.3 Histological Features

The causative organism is a gram-positive, budding, yeast-like cell with an extremely thick, gelatinous capsule. The cryptococcus measures 5–20 μm in diameter and, in tissue sections, appears as small organisms with a large clear halo, sometimes described as "*tissue microcyst*." The capsule is colored intensely with the periodic acid-Schiff (PAS) stain and the organisms may be cultured on Sabouraud's glucose agar.

The tissue reaction is essentially a granulomatous one of the tuberculoid type, but focal necrosis is often absent and epithelioid cell proliferation is minimal. Multinucleated giant cells are common, as is a chronic or subacute inflammatory cell infiltrate. The organisms with their characteristic halo are found singly or in groups scattered throughout the granuloma.

31.4 Treatment and Prognosis

The use of amphotericin B has been found to give excellent results. The ultimate prognosis of patient is variable and especially dependent upon the sites of involvement.

Mucormycosis

32

(Zygomycosis, Phycomycosis)

Contents

32.1	Clinical Features	149
32.2	Radiographic Features	150
32.3	Differential Diagnosis	151
32.4	Histopathologic Features	151
32.5	Treatment and Prognosis	151

Mucormycosis is an opportunistic, frequently fulminant, fungal infection that is caused by normally saprobic organisms of the class Zygomycetes. These organisms are found throughout the world, growing in their natural state on a variety of decaying organic materials. Numerous spores may be liberated into the air and inhaled by the human host.

Mucormycosis may involve any of several areas of the body, but the rhinocerebral form is most relevant to the oral healthcare provider. Mucormycosis is noted especially in insulin-dependent diabetics who have uncontrolled diabetes and are ketoacidotic. This infection affects immunocompromised patients; only rarely has mucormycosis been reported in apparently healthy individuals.

32.1 Clinical Features

The presenting symptoms of rhinocerebral zygomycosis may be exhibited in several ways. Patients may experience nasal obstruction, bloody nasal discharge, facial pain or headache, facial swelling or cellulitis, and visual disturbances with concurrent proptosis. Symptoms related to cranial nerve involvement (e.g., facial paralysis) are often present. With progression of disease into the cranial vault blindness, lethargy and seizures may develop, followed by death.

If the maxillary sinus is involved, the initial presentation may be seen as intraoral swelling of the maxillary alveolar process, the palate, or both. If the condition

© The Author(s), under exclusive license to Springer Nature Singapore Pte Ltd. 2024

K. Paiwal et al., *Handbook of Oral and Maxillofacial Giant Cell Lesions*, https://doi.org/10.1007/978-981-97-2863-3_32

remains untreated, palatal ulceration may evolve, with the surface of the ulcer typically appearing black and necrotic. Massive tissue destruction may result if the condition is not treated.

32.2 Radiographic Features

Varying degrees of soft tissue density occupying the paranasal sinuses can be observed. Linear or wispy, hazy radiopacities can be seen within the soft tissue mass, which represent fungal hyphae. The borders of the sinuses may be destroyed with the lesion invading the nasal cavity or the hard palate, extending into the oral cavity (Fig. 32.1).

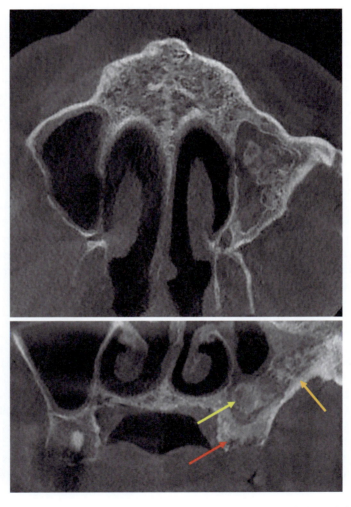

Fig. 32.1 CBCT axial and coronal images showing radiopaque entities within the left maxillary sinus (yellow arrow) along with severe thickening of the mucosa. Note the sclerosis of the sinus walls (orange arrow) and the lesion extending into the alveolar process (red arrow)

32.3 Differential Diagnosis

The differential diagnosis includes benign or malignant neoplasms or infection. Clinical correlation, advanced imaging, and endoscopy may be needed to differentiate between them.

32.4 Histopathologic Features

Histopathologic examination of lesional tissue shows extensive necrosis with numerous large (6–30 μm in diameter), branching, nonseptate hyphae at the periphery. The hyphae tend to branch at 90-degree angles. The extensive tissue destruction and necrosis associated with this disease are undoubtedly attributable to the preference of the fungi for invasion of small blood vessels. This disrupts normal blood flow to the tissue, resulting in infarction and necrosis.

A neutrophil infiltrate is typical and a granulomatous reaction may be observed. This granulomatous infection consists of a chronic exudate of mononuclear cells, histiocytes, epithelioid cells, giant cells, and others admixed with connective tissue.

32.5 Treatment and Prognosis

Treatment of mucormycosis consists of radical surgical debridement of the infected, necrotic tissue and systemic administration of high doses of amphotericin B. Despite such therapy, the prognosis is usually poor.

Aspergillosis

33

Contents

33.1	Clinical Features	153
33.2	Oral Manifestations	154
33.3	Histopathologic Features	154
33.4	Treatment and Prognosis	154

Aspergillosis is a fungal disease that is characterized by noninvasive and invasive forms. Noninvasive aspergillosis usually affects a normal host, appearing either as an allergic reaction or a cluster of fungal hyphae. Localized invasive infection of damaged tissue may be seen in a normal host, but a more extensive invasive infection is often evident in the immunocompromised patient.

Normally, the various species of the *Aspergillus* genus reside worldwide as saprobic organisms in soil, water, or decaying organic debris. Resistant spores are released into the air and inhaled by the human host, resulting in opportunistic fungal infection second in frequency only to candidiasis. Interestingly, most species of *Aspergillus* cannot grow at 37 °C; only the pathogenic species have the ability to replicate at body temperature.

The two most commonly encountered species of aspergillus in the medical setting are *A. flavus* and *A. fumigatus*, with *A. fumigatus* being responsible for 90% of the cases of aspergillosis. The patient may acquire such infections in the hospital (nosocomial infection).

33.1 Clinical Features

The clinical manifestations of aspergillosis vary, depending on the host immune status and the presence or absence of tissue damage. In the normal host, the disease may appear as an allergy affecting either the sinuses (allergic fungal sinusitis) or the

© The Author(s), under exclusive license to Springer Nature Singapore Pte Ltd. 2024
K. Paiwal et al., *Handbook of Oral and Maxillofacial Giant Cell Lesions*, https://doi.org/10.1007/978-981-97-2863-3_33

bronchopulmonary tract. An asthma attack may be triggered by inhalation of spores by a susceptible person. Sometimes a low-grade infection becomes established in the maxillary sinus, resulting in a mass of fungal hyphae called an aspergilloma. Occasionally, the mass undergoes dystrophic calcification, producing a radiopaque body called an enterolith within the sinus.

33.2   Oral Manifestations

The presentation that may be encountered by the oral healthcare provider is aspergillosis after tooth extraction or endodontic treatment, especially in the maxillary posterior segments. Presumably, tissue damage predisposes the sinus to infection, resulting in symptoms of localized pain and tenderness accompanied by nasal discharge. Immunocompromised patients are particularly susceptible to oral aspergillosis, and some investigators have suggested that the portal of entry may be the marginal gingiva and gingival sulcus. Painful gingival ulcerations are initially noted and peripherally the mucosa and soft tissue develop diffuse swelling with a gray or violaceous hue. If the disease is not treated, extensive necrosis, seen clinically as a yellow or black ulcer, and facial swelling evolve. Disseminated aspergillosis occurs principally in immunocompromised patients.

33.3   Histopathologic Features

Tissue sections of aspergillus lesions show varying numbers of branching, septate hyphae, 3–4 μm in diameter. These hyphae show a tendency to branch at an acute angle and to invade adjacent small blood vessels. Occlusion of the vessels often results in the characteristic pattern of necrosis associated with this disease. In the immunocompetent host, a granulomatous inflammatory response in addition to necrosis can be expected. In the immunocompromised patient, the inflammatory response is often weak or absent, leading to extensive tissue destruction.

Aspergillus granuloma shows abundant fibrosis, ill-defined epithelioid granuloma, and many foreign body and Langhans-type giant cells. There is no caseation necrosis. Many giant cells show the presence of fungal fragments within their cytoplasm.

33.4   Treatment and Prognosis

Treatment depends on the clinical presentation of aspergillosis. For immunocompetent patients with a noninvasive aspergilloma, surgical debridement is necessary. Patients who have allergic fungal sinusitis are treated with debridement and corticosteroids. For localized invasive aspergillosis in the immunocompetent host, debridement is indicated. This may be combined with either itraconazole or systemic amphotericin B therapy, depending on the severity of the infection.

The prognosis for immunocompromised patients is much worse compared with immunocompetent individuals, particularly if the infection is disseminated.

Wegener's Granulomatosis

34

Contents

34.1 Etiology... 155
34.2 Clinical Features... 156
34.3 Oral Manifestations.. 156
34.4 Differential Diagnosis... 157
34.5 Histological Features.. 157
34.6 Laboratory Findings.. 157
34.7 Treatment and Prognosis.. 158
Reference... 158

Wegener's granulomatosis (WG) is a rare multisystem disease. In 1931, Klinger first classified WG as a variant of polyarteritis nodosa. In 1936, Wegener described the disease as a distinct entity with specific clinical and histopathologic criteria. The initial description of the syndrome by Wegner included necrotizing granulomatous lesions of the respiratory tract, necrotizing glomerulonephritis, and systemic vasculitis of small arteries and veins.

34.1 Etiology

The specific cause of WG is unknown. Analysis of bronchoalveolar lavage in recently diagnosed patients revealed no evidence of specific bacteria, fungi, or viruses. Although this does not fully rule out an infectious agent as the cause of WG, it does suggest that, if present, the agent is there for a very short period of time and/or cannot be detected by current laboratory techniques.

© The Author(s), under exclusive license to Springer Nature Singapore Pte Ltd. 2024
K. Paiwal et al., *Handbook of Oral and Maxillofacial Giant Cell Lesions*,
https://doi.org/10.1007/978-981-97-2863-3_34

Some investigators believe that this disease is caused by an abnormal immune reaction secondary to a nonspecific infection or a hypersensitivity reaction to an unknown antigen. A possible hereditary predisposition has been mentioned in some cases.

34.2 Clinical Features

Wegener's granulomatosis may occur at any age, from infants to the very elderly, although the majority of cases are in the fourth and fifth decades of life. There is a slight predilection for occurrence in males.

Akikusa et al. [1] in their study observed a significant female predominance, with a male to female ratio of 1:4.

The prevalence of the disease has been reported to be 3.0 per 100,000. The disease can involve almost every organ system in the body. With classic Wegener's granulomatosis, patients initially show involvement of the upper and lower respiratory tract; if the condition remains untreated, renal involvement often rapidly develops. Limited Wegener's granulomatosis is diagnosed when there is involvement of the respiratory system without rapid development of renal lesions. One subset of patients exhibits lesions primarily of the skin and mucosa, a condition termed superficial Wegener's granulomatosis. In this form of the disease, systemic involvement develops slowly. These three different clinical patterns highlight the variability of the clinical aggressiveness that can occur in patients with Wegner's granulomatosis.

Purulent nasal discharge, chronic sinus pain, nasal ulceration, congestion, and fever are frequent findings from upper respiratory involvement. Persistent otitis media, sore throat, and epistaxis also are reported. With progression, destruction of the nasal septum can result in a saddle nose deformity. Patients with lower respiratory involvement may be asymptomatic or they may have dry cough, hemoptysis, and dyspnea or chest pain.

Renal involvement usually occurs late in the disease process and is the most frequent cause of death. The glomerulonephritis results in proteinuria and red blood cell casts. Occasionally, the eyes, ears, and skin also are involved.

34.3 Oral Manifestations

Involvement of the oral cavity occurs with considerable frequency in WG. However, only rarely the oral lesions are the first manifestation of the disease.

The most characteristic oral manifestation is strawberry gingivitis. This distinctive but uncommon pattern of gingival alteration appears to be an early manifestation of WG and occurs before renal involvement in most cases. The affected gingiva demonstrates a florid and granular hyperplasia. The surface forms numerous short bulbous projections, which are hemorrhagic and friable. The buccal surfaces are affected more frequently and the alterations are classically confined to the attached gingiva.

The inflammatory process starts in the interdental papilla and spreads rapidly to the periodontal structure. This leads to bone loss and tooth mobility.

Oral ulceration also may be a manifestation of WG. These are clinically nonspecific and may occur on any mucosal surface. These are diagnosed at a later stage of the disease. Other less common orofacial manifestations include facial paralysis, labial mucosal nodules, sinusitis-related toothache, arthralgia of the TMJ, jaw claudication, palatal ulceration from nasal extension, oral-antral fistulae, and poorly healing extraction sites. Enlargement of one or more major salivary glands has been reported. The glandular involvement appears in the early course of the disease.

34.4 Differential Diagnosis

Nasopharynx involvement is difficult to differentiate from sinonasal lymphoma or sarcoidosis on imaging.

34.5 Histological Features

Wegener's granulomatosis appears as a pattern of mixed inflammation centered around blood vessels. Involved vessels demonstrate transmural inflammation, often with areas of heavy neutrophilic infiltration, necrosis, and nuclear dust (leukocytoclastic vasculitis). The connective tissue adjacent to the vessel has an inflammatory cellular infiltrate, which contains a variable mixture of histiocytes, lymphocytes, eosinophils, and multinucleated giant cells. Special stains for organism are negative and no foreign material can be found.

In oral biopsy specimens, the oral epithelium may demonstrate pseudoepitheliomatous hyperplasia and subepithelial abscesses. Because of the paucity of large vessels in many oral mucosal biopsies, vasculitis may be difficult to demonstrate, and the histopathologic presentation may be one of the ill-defined collections of epithelioid histiocytes intermixed with lymphocytes, eosinophils, and multinucleated giant cells.

The lesions of strawberry gingivitis typically demonstrate prominent vascularity with extensive red blood cell extravasation.

34.6 Laboratory Findings

Laboratory findings include anemia, leukocytosis, ESR, and hyperglobulinemia. Because of kidney involvement, hematuria is common along with the finding of albumin, casts, and leukocytes in the urine.

Indirect immunofluorescence for serum antibodies directed against cytoplasmic components of neutrophils has been used to support a diagnosis of WG. There are two reaction patterns of these antineutrophil cytoplasmic antibodies (ANCA):

1. Perinuclear (p-ANCA)
2. Cytoplasmic (c-ANCA)

Cytoplasmic localization (c-ANCA) is most useful and is present in 90–95% of cases of acute generalized WG. This positivity drops to 60% in early localized form of the disease. When positive, a finding of c-ANCA confirms the diagnosis.

34.7 Treatment and Prognosis

The mean survival of untreated patients with disseminated classic WG is 5 months; 80% of the patients die in 1 year and 90% within 2 years. However, the prognosis is better for the limited and superficial forms of the disease.

The drugs of choice are cyclophosphamide and prednisone but have serious potential side effects. Trimethoprim-sulfamethoxazole has been used successfully in localized cases and when the immunosuppressive regimen has failed. Low-dose methotrexate and corticosteroids also have been used in patients whose disease is not immediately life-threatening. New treatment options under study include cyclo-sporine and intravenous pooled immunoglobulin.

Reference

1. Akikusa JD, Schneider R, Harvey EA, Hebert D, Thorner PS, Laxer RM, Silverman ED. Clinical features and outcome of pediatric Wegener's granulomatosis. Arthritis Rheum. 2007;57(5):837–44.

Periapical Pathosis

35

Contents

35.1 Periapical Granuloma 159
35.2 Histopathology 160
35.3 Periapical Cyst 160
35.4 Histopathologic Features 160
35.5 Treatment 160
35.6 Radiographic Features of Periapical Pathosis 161
35.7 Differential Diagnosis 162

Numerous sequelae may follow untreated pulp necrosis. These are dependent on the virulence of the microorganisms involved and the integrity of the patient's overall defense mechanisms. From its origin in the pulp, the inflammatory process extends into the periapical tissues, where it may present as a granuloma or cyst (if chronic) or an abscess (if acute). Acute exacerbation of a chronic lesion may also be seen. The necrotic pulpal tissue debris, inflammatory cells, and bacteria, particularly anaerobes, all serve to stimulate and sustain the periapical inflammatory process.

35.1 Periapical Granuloma

Periapical granuloma is a low-grade infection and is essentially a localized mass of chronic granulation tissue formed in response to the infection.

The involved tooth is usually non-vital and may be slightly tender to percussion. Percussion may produce a dull sound instead of a normal metallic sound because of the presence of granulation tissue around the root apex. Patients may complain about mild pain from biting or chewing on solid food. In some cases, the tooth feels slightly elongated in its socket. The sensitivity is due to hyperemia, edema, and inflammation of the apical periodontal ligament.

© The Author(s), under exclusive license to Springer Nature Singapore Pte Ltd. 2024
K. Paiwal et al., *Handbook of Oral and Maxillofacial Giant Cell Lesions*,
https://doi.org/10.1007/978-981-97-2863-3_35

35.2 Histopathology

A periapical granuloma is composed of an outer capsule of dense fibrous tissue and a central zone of granulation tissue. The central zone will often contain macrophages with a *foamy* cytoplasm caused by phagocytized cholesterol. Some cholesterol crystals may be present, surrounded by multinucleated giant cells of the foreign body type. Throughout, the soft tissue will be a diffuse infiltrate of lymphocytes and plasma cells. Irregular islands and strands of epithelium are also present which are a result of prolonged, mild stimulation of the *rests of Malassez*.

35.3 Periapical Cyst

A periapical cyst is a common development of long-standing, untreated periapical granuloma. The cyst's epithelial lining is derived from the cell rests of Malassez. The rests are stimulated to proliferate by the low-grade inflammation of the preceding periapical granuloma.

The majority of cases are asymptomatic and present no clinical evidence of their presence. They are commonly seen between the ages of 20 and 60 years, but the involvement of deciduous dentition is not uncommon. The most commonly involved teeth are maxillary anteriors. The associated tooth is non-vital or shows deep carious lesion or a restoration which is seldom painful or even sensitive to percussion. The cyst is only infrequently of such a size that it destroys much bone and rarely produces expansion of the cortical plate.

35.4 Histopathologic Features

The tissue consists of an outer dense fibrous connective tissue capsule that surrounds a central lumen containing a thick, proteinaceous fluid and cellular debris. The lumen is lined by a nonkeratinized, stratified squamous epithelium containing rete pegs that are generally elongated and branched. Collections of cholesterol-laden macrophages are commonly present, particularly in the early stages of cyst development. The capsule and the epithelial lining contain a diffuse infiltration of plasma cells and lymphocytes. Cholesterol crystals surrounded by foreign body giant cells are a common finding. The presence of eosinophilic refractile hyaline bodies, referred to as *Rushton bodies*, is sometimes found in the intermediate cell layer of the epithelium.

35.5 Treatment

If the tooth is restorable, the root canal can be filled; otherwise, the tooth is extracted.

35.6 Radiographic Features of Periapical Pathosis

Radiographically, it is not possible to differentiate the various periapical pathoses such as periapical granuloma, abscess, or cyst. So, they are grouped under the term "rarefying osteitis." It is only after histopathologic examination that periapical cysts can be determined with certainty. The radiographic features of periapical inflammatory lesions vary depending on stage of the lesion. Early at onset, the affected tooth might not show any change at all radiographically or demonstrate very subtle changes. As the lesion progresses, periapical radiolucency might become evident which may or may be surrounded by a zone of sclerosis (Fig. 35.1). The margins are usually poorly defined but well localized with a narrow to wide zone of transition to the normal bone. At times, in long-standing cases, the margins might be well-defined with corticated borders, more suggestive of a cyst (Fig. 35.2). The affected teeth will lose the lamina dura in the apical region along with widening of the periodontal ligament space. If the lesions are adjacent to the floor of the maxillary sinus, there might be localized thickening of the mucosal lining within the sinus.

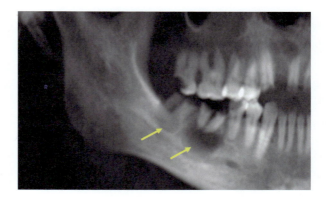

Fig. 35.1 Cropped panoramic image showing well-defined periapical radiolucent lesions associated with grossly carious right mandibular molars (yellow arrows)

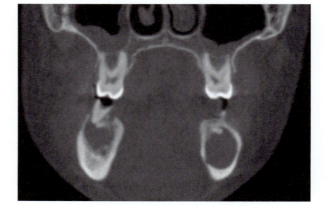

Fig. 35.2 CBCT coronal section showing well-defined periapical radiolucent lesions associated with grossly carious mandibular teeth bilaterally. The right-side lesion also shows areas of sclerosis within the entity depicting chronicity of the lesion

35.7 Differential Diagnosis

1. **Periapical scar:** The periapical fibrous healing associated with endodontically treated tooth may appear similar to a periapical infection. Correlating with clinical findings, and comparing with previous radiographs, if available, would help in differentiating the entities.
2. **Periapical osseous dysplasia:** Here the involved teeth would be vital. Mostly seen in the mandibular anterior region with multiple teeth involved. The periodontal ligament space appears intact.
3. **Malignant and metastatic lesions:** Rarely, these malignancies mimic periapical pathosis. Irregular widening of the periodontal ligament space is a diagnostic clue for malignancy. Also, the lesions occur without any source of infection.

Giant Cell Fibroma

36

Contents

36.1	Clinical Features	163
36.2	Histological Features	163
36.3	Treatment and Prognosis	164
Reference		164

Giant cell fibroma (GCF) is a benign nonneoplastic lesion first described by Weathers and Callihan [1]. The GCF is a fibrous tumor with distinctive clinico-pathological features. Unlike the traumatic fibroma, it does not appear to be associated with chronic irritation. The giant cell fibroma represents approximately 2–5% of all oral fibrous proliferations submitted for biopsy.

36.1 Clinical Features

Giant cell fibroma occurs in the first three decades of life and predominates in females. The GCF is typically an asymptomatic sessile or pedunculated nodule, usually <1 cm in size. The surface of the mass often appears papillary; therefore, the lesion may be clinically mistaken for a papilloma. Approximately 50% of all the cases occur on the gingiva. The mandibular gingiva is affected twice as often as the maxillary gingiva. The tongue and palate are also common sites.

36.2 Histological Features

Microscopically, a giant cell fibroma is an unencapsulated mass of loose fibrous connective tissue. The connective tissue contains numerous characteristic large, plump, spindle-shaped, and stellate fibroblasts, some of which are multinucleated.

© The Author(s), under exclusive license to Springer Nature Singapore Pte Ltd. 2024
K. Paiwal et al., *Handbook of Oral and Maxillofacial Giant Cell Lesions*, https://doi.org/10.1007/978-981-97-2863-3_36

These cells are easily observed in the peripheral areas of the lesion, whereas the more central area contains typical fusiform fibroblasts. The surface epithelium is corrugated and atrophic; in contrast to an irritation fibroma, a giant cell fibroma has a thin, elongated rete ridge.

The origin of stellate and multinucleated cells is not well known. Few studies showed positive immunostaining for vimentin. This suggests that the stellate and multinucleated cells of GCF have a fibroblast phenotype.

36.3 Treatment and Prognosis

Conservative excisional biopsy is curative and its findings are diagnostic. Recurrence is rare.

Reference

1. Weathers DR, Callihan MD. Giant-cell fibroma. Oral Surg Oral Med Oral Pathol. 1974;37(3):374–84. https://doi.org/10.1016/0030-4220(74)90110-8. PMID: 4521457.

Traumatic Granuloma

37

(Eosinophilic Ulceration, Traumatic Ulcerative Granuloma with Stromal Eosinophilia [TUGSE])

Contents

37.1 Clinical Features.. 165
37.2 Histological Features... 166
37.3 Treatment and Prognosis... 166

Acute or chronic trauma to the oral mucosa may result in surface ulcerations. The ulcerations may remain for extended periods of time but most usually heal within days. These exhibit a deep pseudo invasive inflammatory reaction and are typically slow to resolve.

In addition, similar sublingual ulcerations may occur in infants as a result of chronic mucosal trauma from adjacent primary anterior teeth, often associated with nursing. These distinctive ulcerations of infancy have been termed Riga-Fede disease and are a variation of the traumatic eosinophilic ulceration.

In most cases of traumatic ulceration, there is an adjacent source of irritation, although this is not present invariably. The clinical presentation often suggests the cause, but many cases resemble early ulcerative squamous cell carcinoma; biopsy is performed to rule out that possibility.

37.1 Clinical Features

Traumatic granuloma (TG) is commonly observed in all age groups, with a significant male predominance. They are usually seen in the anteroventral and dorsal surfaces of the tongue. Lesions may also be observed in other sites such as the gingiva, the palate, and the mucobuccal fold.

Traumatic granuloma is a chronic, benign, self-limiting lesion of the oral mucosa, manifesting as an ulcer with elevated margins. The ulcerations usually persist up to

© The Author(s), under exclusive license to Springer Nature Singapore Pte Ltd. 2024
K. Paiwal et al., *Handbook of Oral and Maxillofacial Giant Cell Lesions*, https://doi.org/10.1007/978-981-97-2863-3_37

a week or even up to 8 months. They resemble the simple traumatic ulcerations, appearing as areas of erythema surrounding a central removable yellow fibrinopurulent membrane. Further, rolled borders of hyperorthokeratosis may develop immediately adjacent to the area of ulceration. The proliferation of the underlying granulation tissue can lead to a raised lesion resembling pyogenic granuloma.

37.2 Histological Features

Simple traumatic ulcerations are covered by a fibrinopurulent membrane that consists of fibrin intermixed with neutrophils. The membrane is of variable thickness. The adjacent surface epithelium may be normal or may demonstrate slight hyperplasia with or without hyperkeratosis.

Microscopically, traumatic granuloma is characterized by a dense polymorphic inflammatory infiltrate extending into the underlying muscle. The dominant cell types in the inflammatory infiltrate are small lymphocytes, with abundant eosinophils.

Mucosal degeneration is characteristic and may be attributed to proliferation of cytotoxic T cells or toxic products released by degranulating eosinophils. This degenerated mucosa permits the ingress of microorganisms, toxins, and foreign proteins into the connective tissue. In predisposed persons, these substances induce a severe inflammatory response resulting from an exaggerated mast cell-eosinophil reaction similar to that noticed in the pathogenesis of bronchial asthma.

The presence of large, atypical mononuclear cell is another microscopic feature of TG present in most cases. The origin of these large cells has been a matter of debate. Some scientists believe them to be of macrophage origin and some say that they represent myofibroblasts.

37.3 Treatment and Prognosis

For traumatic ulcerations that have an obvious source of injury, the irritating cause should be removed. If the cause is not obvious or if a patient does not respond to therapy, biopsy is indicated. Rapid healing after a biopsy is typical even with large eosinophilic ulcerations. Recurrence is not expected.

Solitary Bone Cyst

38

(Traumatic Bone Cyst, Simple Bone Cyst, Hemorrhagic Bone Cyst, Extravasation Cyst, Unicameral Bone Cyst, Idiopathic Bone Cyst)

Contents

38.1	Clinical Features	168
38.2	Radiographic Features	168
38.3	Differential Diagnosis	169
38.4	Histological Features	169
38.5	Treatment	169
References		169

The simple bone cyst was first described by Lucas in 1929. Since then, it has been reported in various articles under a variety of names, i.e., solitary bone cyst, hemorrhagic bone cyst, traumatic bone cyst, extravasation bone cyst, idiopathic bone cavity, and progressive bone cavity, as there was no unanimous agreement on the exact nature and the probable cause of the cyst.

Rushton [1] defined it as a vacant or fluid-containing cystic lesion surrounded by a hard bony wall with no epithelial lining and no evidence of infection.

The international histologic classification of tumors by WHO recommended the use of the term solitary bone cyst in 1992.

The traumatic bone cyst is a benign empty or fluid-containing cavity within the bone that is devoid of an epithelial lining. Although a solitary bone cyst is an intraosseous empty cavity, it is sometimes lined by a thin layer of fibrous connective tissue without epithelium. It can also contain serosanguinous fluid, granulation tissue, erythrocytes, hemosiderin, and osteoclast.

A solitary bone cyst is an anatomic indentation of the posterior lingual mandible that appears to resemble a cyst on radiographic examination. This depression of the mandible is believed to be developmental in origin. It is an unusual benign, empty, or fluid-filled cavity within bone that is devoid of epithelial lining.

© The Author(s), under exclusive license to Springer Nature Singapore Pte Ltd. 2024

K. Paiwal et al., *Handbook of Oral and Maxillofacial Giant Cell Lesions*, https://doi.org/10.1007/978-981-97-2863-3_38

38.1 Clinical Features

The solitary bone cyst is not a common lesion. This cystic lesion is usually asymptomatic and is discovered during routine radiographic examination. In some cases, enlargement of the mandible, most frequently buccal and labial, can be seen.

Howe [2] used the following criteria to determine the cases; cyst should be single, have no epithelial lining, and show no evidence of acute or prolonged infection. It should contain principally fluid and not soft tissue. The walls should be of bone which is hard although possibly thin in parts.

The simple bone cyst occurs in young individuals. The patients ranged in age from 25 to 35 years. Killey et al. [3] recorded a peak frequency in the second decade. Male to female ratio is 1.6:1 and majority of lesions occur in mandible. Almost all the maxillary cases involve the anterior regions and the majority of the mandibular cases have been reported in the body and symphyseal area. In some cases, enlargement of the mandible has been observed.

The pulps of the teeth in the involved area are vital and do not show root resorption. When the cavity is opened surgically, it is found to contain either a small amount of straw-colored fluid, shreds of necrotic clot, fragments of fibrous connective tissue, or nothing.

38.2 Radiographic Features

Simple bone cyst usually appears as a well-defined, unilocular radiolucency with subtle corticated borders (Fig. 38.1). Because of the delicate nature, the cortication may be easily missed. The borders are less clear inferiorly than superiorly. In the teeth-bearing areas, the borders tend to scallop around the roots of the teeth. Sometimes, they appear to septa but this appearance is due the pronounced scalloping of the cortical borders. These lesions tend to grow along the long axis of the

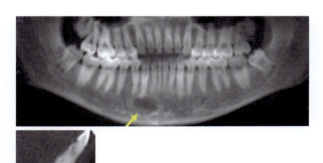

Fig. 38.1 Reconstructed panoramic radiograph and cropped sagittal views showing a well-defined, corticated, unilocular hypodense in the right mandibular anterior region (yellow arrow). Thinning of the lingual border of the mandible is noted (white arrow). Lamina dura of the adjacent teeth is intact (orange arrow). (Courtesy AZ. Syed, BDS, MHA, MS, Dipl. ABOMR)

bone causing little or no expansion of the cortices. When observed closely, the lamina dura of the involved teeth is preserved. Rarely, minor displacement or resorption of the teeth may be seen.

38.3 Differential Diagnosis

1. **Odontogenic keratocyst:** Occurs in older age groups. Grows along bone with minimal expansion and scalloped borders similar to SBC. However, KOT usually has a more definite cortical boundary.
2. **Odontogenic myxoma:** Causes minimal expansion and scalloped borders similar to SBC. However, straight and fine septa are characteristic for this lesion.

38.4 Histological Features

The simple bone cyst consists of a thin, loose vascular fibrous tissue membrane of variable thickness with no epithelial lining or demonstrates a thickened myxofibromatous proliferation that is often intermixed with trabeculae of cellular and reactive bone. Hemorrhage and hemosiderin pigment are usually present and scattered small multinucleated giant cells are often found. Some cyst walls, possibly cases of long standing, are more densely fibrous.

The adjacent bone, when included in the specimen, shows osteoclastic resorption (Howship's lacunae) on its inner surface. Beasley [4] described areas of hemorrhage associated with necrotic tissue or tissue showing myxoid degeneration. These occurred in cavities adjacent to areas of bone resorption. Thrombi were not observed in any of the specimens which he examined. Cases associated with florid osseous dysplasia or cemento-osseous dysplasias have been reported.

38.5 Treatment

Simple surgical exploration to establish the diagnosis is usually sufficient therapy for solitary bone cyst of jaws. After surgical exploration with or without curettage of the bony walls, obliteration of the defect by new bone formation is generally rapid. Recurrence or persistence of the lesion is most unusual. The prognosis is, however, excellent.

References

1. Rushton MA. Solitary bone cysts in the mandible. Br Dent J. 1946;81(2):37–49. PMID: 20992458.
2. Howe GL. 'Haemorrhagic cysts' of the mandible. Br J Oral Surg. 1965;3:55–76.
3. Killey HC, Kay LW, Seward GR. Benign cystic lesions of the jaws, their diagnosis and treatment. 3rd ed. Edinburgh: Churchill Livingstone; 1977.
4. Beasley JD. Traumatic cyst of the jaws: report of 30 cases. J Am Dent Assoc. 1976;92:145–52.

Osteoid Osteoma

39

Contents

39.1 Clinical Features. ... 171
39.2 Oral Features. ... 172
39.3 Radiographic Features. ... 172
39.4 Differential Diagnosis. ... 173
39.5 Histopathologic Features. ... 174
39.6 Treatment and Prognosis. ... 174

Osteoid osteoma is a benign, solitary, painful circumscribed osteoblastic bone tumor of spongy bone. It was first identified as a clinical entity by Jaffe in 1935. It has been shown that the tumor nidus in osteoid osteomas contains a concentration of peripheral nerves not seen in other fibro-osseous neoplasms. Jaffe and Lichtenstein have suggested that the lesion is a true neoplasm of osteoblastic derivation, but others have suggested that the lesion occurs as a result of trauma or inflammation. In some instances, it can be confused with osteomyelitis and may actually represent a form of osteomyelitis. The size of osteoid osteoma is <2 cm. Osteoid osteoma and osteoblastoma are closely related benign bone tumors, with osteoid osteoma being under 2 cm and osteoblastoma being larger than 2 cm.

39.1 Clinical Features

Osteoid osteoma usually occurs in the second and third decades of life. Men are affected more frequently than women having male to female ratio of at least 2:1. Osteoid osteomas occur most often in the femur, tibia, and phalanges. They are very

© The Author(s), under exclusive license to Springer Nature Singapore Pte Ltd. 2024

K. Paiwal et al., *Handbook of Oral and Maxillofacial Giant Cell Lesions*, https://doi.org/10.1007/978-981-97-2863-3_39

rare in the jaws but if they occur, there is mandibular predominance. The body of the mandible is affected in most of the cases. They can be classified as cortical, cancellous, and subperiosteal depending on the position of the lesion.

The lesion consists of a small radiolucent nidus containing nerve fibers, vascular elements, and very high levels of prostaglandin which causes chronic reactive change in the surrounding bone resulting in marked surrounding periosteal sclerosis and synovitis. The excess sclerotic bone helps to point the location of the lesion during surgery. The prostaglandin is responsible for the constant, severe pain which is the most common presenting symptom.

Pain is severe, unrelenting, and sharp which is worse at night. It is usually nocturnal in nature and alleviated by salicylates like aspirin. Localized swelling of the soft tissue over the involved area of the bone may occur and may be tender.

39.2 Oral Features

Very few cases of osteoid osteomas have been reported occurring in the jaws. In the seven cases that have been reported, four have occurred in the mandible (three in body; one in condyle) and one in maxilla (maxillary antrum).

39.3 Radiographic Features

Radiographically, the osteoid osteoma appears as a predominantly radiopaque entity with a central radiolucent nidus. The lesion is usually well circumscribed. The central nidus may sometimes exhibit radiopaque foci. The overlying cortex becomes thickened by subperiosteal new bone formation. This all results in a target-like appearance radiographically (Fig. 39.1).

Fig. 39.1 Axial and coronal CBCT images showing a well-defined, pedunculated, and lobulated, radiopaque entity emerging from the medial aspect of the left mandibular angle (yellow arrows). (Courtesy R. Alansari, BDS)

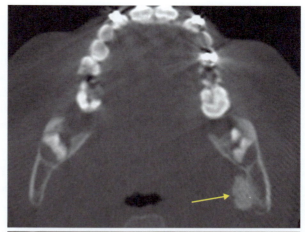
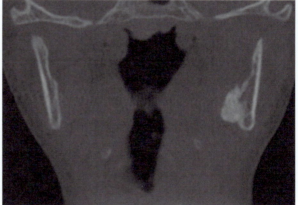

39.4 Differential Diagnosis

1. **Osteoblastoma:** Less painful. This pain is not relieved by nonsteroidal anti-inflammatory medication. More aggressive with greater growth potential.
2. **Cemento-ossifying fibroma:** Concentric growth pattern, has thin, radiolucent rim (fibrous capsule), painless.
3. **Cementoblastoma:** Occurs around root apex (mostly lower first molar), causes root resorption, has a wheel spoke pattern.
4. **Periapical osseous dysplasia:** Usually multifocal and painless. Occurs in the mandibular anterior region.
5. **Periapical sclerosing osteitis:** Associated with a non-vital tooth, loss of lamina dura, and widened periodontal ligament space.

39.5 Histopathologic Features

The histological appearance of osteoid osteoma is characteristic. It consists of a central nidus which is composed of compact osteoid tissue, varying in degree of calcification, interspersed by a vascular connective tissue. There is definite trabeculae formation which occurs mainly in older lesions. These trabeculae are lined by osteoblasts. New bone formation occurs in the overlying periosteum. Osteoclasts and foci of bone resorption may be seen. Interstitial tissue collections of lymphocytes may also be present.

Ultrastructurally, morphology of osteoblasts is similar to that of normal osteoblasts except for the mitochondria which is atypical. The morphology of osteoid osteoma is almost similar to that of osteoblastoma including atypical mitochondria. The difference between them is that in osteoid osteoma, neutral staining techniques reveal many axons throughout the nidus which probably account for pain. Levels of prostaglandin E_2 are markedly elevated in the nidus which causes vasodilatation and results in further aggravation of pain.

39.6 Treatment and Prognosis

Most cases of osteoid osteoma are treated by local excision of the lesion or curettage. The prognosis is good but a few lesions regress after incomplete excision.

Osteoblastoma

(Giant Osteoid Osteoma)

40

Contents

40.1	Clinical Features.	175
40.2	Radiographic Features.	176
40.3	Differential Diagnosis.	177
40.4	Histological Features.	177
40.5	Treatment and Prognosis.	177
References.		178

Osteoblastoma is a benign, vascular, and progressively expansile tumor of the bone. It is an uncommon lesion that accounts for 1% of all bone tumors and about 3% of all benign bone tumors.

The osteoblastic nature of the tumor often results in zones similar to those of an osteoid osteoma producing a histological resemblance. Benign osteoblastoma differs, however, in that it does not share the markedly limited growth potential of the average osteoid osteoma. Furthermore, the benign osteoblastoma frequently lacks the characteristic pain and the halo of sclerotic bone associated with osteoid osteoma. The size of the osteoblastoma is also more than 1.5 cm in its greatest dimension.

The benign osteoblastoma was first described under the name "giant osteoid osteoma" by Dahlin and Johnson [1] and under the presently more accepted name by Jaffe and by Lichtenstein in 1956.

40.1 Clinical Features

Osteoblastoma occurs most frequently in young persons, approximately 90% under 30 years of age. However, it does occur even in elderly adults. It occurs more frequently in males (2–3:1). The lesion is characterized by pain and swelling at the tumor site.

© The Author(s), under exclusive license to Springer Nature Singapore Pte Ltd. 2024
K. Paiwal et al., *Handbook of Oral and Maxillofacial Giant Cell Lesions*,
https://doi.org/10.1007/978-981-97-2863-3_40

The most common site of occurrence is the vertebral column. The first case in the jaws was reported by Borello and Sedano [2]. It occurs in both the maxilla and mandible with almost same frequency.

A small group of osteoblastomas (*aggressive osteoblastomas*) is characterized by more atypical histopathologic features and locally aggressive behavior. These tumors usually occur in older patients with most being over 30 years of age.

40.2 Radiographic Features

Osteoblastoma is a predominantly radiopaque entity with a radiolucent rim which is in turn surrounded by a zone of sclerosis or cortication. In early stages, the lesion appears more radiolucent with areas of calcification. In some cases, the margins may be diffuse. Bony expansion is a feature, but a thin outer cortex is always maintained (Fig. 40.1). It may cause displacement of teeth and root resorption if present in the tooth-bearing region.

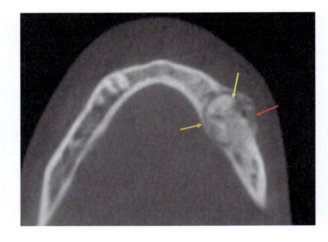

Fig. 40.1 CBCT axial section of a case of osteoblastoma showing a well-defined, mixed density lesion in the left mandibular region (yellow arrow), surrounded by a radiolucent rim (orange arrow). Note the expansion of the buccal cortical plate (red arrow)

40.3 Differential Diagnosis

1. **Osteoid osteoma:** More painful, smaller in size with more sclerotic periphery
2. **Cemento-ossifying fibroma:** Concentric growth pattern, has thin, radiolucent rim (fibrous capsule), painless
3. **Cementoblastoma:** Occurs around root apex, mostly lower first molar, causes root resorption, has a wheel spoke pattern
4. **Periapical osseous dysplasia:** Usually multifocal and painless. Occurs in the mandibular anterior region
5. **Periapical sclerosing osteitis:** Associated with a non-vital tooth, loss of lamina dura, and widened periodontal ligament space

40.4 Histological Features

Histologically, it consists of a highly vascularized, fibro-cellular stroma in which there are abundant newly formed trabeculae of immature bone and osteoid. The mineralized material demonstrates prominent reversal lines. Proliferating osteoblasts are found lining the trabeculae of immature bone and osteoid. At the periphery of the large masses and surrounding the trabeculae are scattered multinucleated osteoclast-like cells. These osteoblasts and osteoclasts have ample cytoplasm and hyperchromatic nuclei.

The supporting stroma consists of loose fibrous connective tissue that contains scattered dilated vascular channels. Focal areas of hemorrhage are common.

Microscopically, aggressive osteoblastomas are characterized by the presence of large epithelioid osteoblasts with increased mitotic activity and non-trabecular sheets or lace-like areas of osteoid production. On occasion, osteoblastomas may demonstrate a rich cellularity that leads to erroneous diagnosis of osteosarcoma.

Malignant transformation (osteosarcoma) within a benign osteoblastoma is very rare. A *malignant osteoblastoma* has been described by Schajowicz and Lemos on the basis of a histologically, i.e., more bizarre pattern of cells, more abundant and often plump hyperchromatic nuclei, greater nuclear atypia, and numerous giant cells. It has a better prognosis than a conventional osteosarcoma.

40.5 Treatment and Prognosis

Most cases of osteoblastoma are treated by local excision or curettage. The prognosis is good, and some lesions will regress even after incomplete excision.

References

1. Dahlin DC, et al. Giant osteoid osteoma. J Bone Joint Surg Am. 1954;36:559.
2. Borello ED, Sedano HO. Giant osteoid osteoma of the maxilla: report of a case. Oral Surg. 1967;23:563.

Radicular Cyst

41

Contents

41.1	Pathogenesis	179
41.2	Clinical Features	180
41.3	Radiographic Features	181
41.4	Histopathologic Features	182
41.5	Differential Diagnosis	183
41.6	Treatment	183
Reference		183

The periapical cyst is a common but inevitable sequela of the periapical granuloma originating as a result of bacterial infection and pulpal necrosis, nearly always following carious involvement of the teeth. The epithelium at the apex of a non-vital tooth can be stimulated by inflammation to form a true epithelium-lined cyst or a periapical cyst.

Occasionally a similar cyst, best termed as the lateral radicular cyst, may appear along the lateral aspect of the root. Periapical inflammatory tissue that is not curetted at the time of tooth removal may give rise to an inflammatory cyst called as the residual periapical cyst. The occurrence of the radicular cyst in deciduous dentition is considered to be rare compared to that in the permanent dentition.

41.1 Pathogenesis

This cyst is almost invariably lined by stratified squamous epithelium, and the wall is made up of condensed connective tissue. The initial reaction leading to a cyst formation is proliferation of the epithelial rests in the periapical area involved by the granuloma. This epithelial proliferation follows an irregular pattern of growth and

---

© The Author(s), under exclusive license to Springer Nature Singapore Pte Ltd. 2024
K. Paiwal et al., *Handbook of Oral and Maxillofacial Giant Cell Lesions*, https://doi.org/10.1007/978-981-97-2863-3_41

occasionally presents a frightening picture because of the pseudo invasiveness and inflammatory appearance of the cells. This proliferation continues with the epithelial mass increasing in size by division of the cells on the periphery, corresponding to the basal layer of the surface epithelium. The cells in the central portion of the mass get separated further from their source of nutrition, the capillaries and tissue fluid of the connective tissue. As these central cells become devoid of sufficient nutrients, they eventually degenerate, become necrotic, and liquefy. This creates an epithelium-lined cavity filled with fluid leading to the periapical cyst.

This cyst may arise also through the proliferation of epithelium lining a pre-existing cavity formed through focal necrosis and degeneration of connective tissue in a periapical granuloma.

Immunological studies have demonstrated the presence of IgG, IgM, IgA, and C3 in these cysts and suggested that both the humoral and cell-mediated immunity may play a role in the pathogenesis of radicular cyst.

41.2 Clinical Features

The majorities of the periapical cysts are asymptomatic and are discovered when periapical radiographs of teeth with non-vital pulps are taken. The tooth is seldom painful or even sensitive to percussion. At first the enlargement is bony hard, but as the cyst increases in size, the covering bone becomes very thin despite subperiosteal bone deposition, and the swelling then exhibits "springiness." When the cyst has completely eroded the bone, there will be fluctuation.

In some cases, the cysts of long-standing duration may undergo acute exacerbation of the inflammatory process and develop rapidly into an abscess that may produce cellulitis or form a fistula.

In the maxilla there may be buccal or palatal enlargement, whereas in the mandible it is usually labial or buccal and rarely lingual. Radicular cysts are painless unless infected. A sine qua non for the diagnosis of a radicular cyst is the presence of a tooth with a non-vital pulp. Occasionally, a sinus may form from the cystic cavity. The tooth from which the cyst originated does not respond to thermal or electric pulp testing.

The frequency of radicular cysts originating from primary teeth as reflected by the number of reported cases is substantially lower than those associated with permanent teeth. In the deciduous teeth, it is more frequently associated with the first molar. Higher incidence of the occurrence of cysts when compared to granulomas in the primary dentition may be due to a large number of epithelial rest cells in the environment of the mixed dentition or due to a high tendency of the epithelial rests to proliferate in the presence of inflammatory irritation.

Mass et al. [1] in their study and review of literature suggested that radicular cysts associated with primary teeth are not rare. They analyzed 49 primary molars with radiolucent lesions ranging from 4 to 15 mm in diameter. 73.5% of the lesions were diagnosed as radicular cyst and 26.5% as granulomas. The lesions were more frequent in the mandible and were associated with severely decayed teeth and with previous pulp therapy.

The mandibular primary teeth are affected more frequently than the maxillary teeth, in contrast to the maxillary predominance in the permanent dentition. The difference in the site distribution can be explained by the fact that in the primary dentition, caries is the frequent etiological factor, and the mandibular molars are the most frequently affected teeth. In the permanent maxillary incisors, the high frequency of radicular cyst results from trauma, caries, and old silicate restorations. Most radicular cysts of the primary dentition are located in the interradicular area and around the roots, because of the short as well as resorbed roots and presence of accessory canals in the primary teeth. Thus, the term "peri-radicular" cyst is more appropriate than periapical cyst in the primary dentition.

41.3 Radiographic Features

The radiographic pattern is identical in most cases to that of a periapical granuloma. The classical radiographic description of a periapical cyst is a well-defined, round or ovoid periapical radiolucency surrounded by corticated margin extending from the lamina dura. Infected or rapidly enlarging cysts may not show the cortication. Lateral radicular cysts appear as discrete radiolucency along the lateral aspect of the root. The residual periapical cyst appears as a round to oval radiolucency of variable size within the alveolar ridge at the site of a previous tooth extraction. As the cyst ages, degeneration of the cellular contents within the lumen occasionally leads to dystrophic calcification and central luminal radiopacity. If the lesions are large, they can cause expansion and thinning of the cortices which may lead to bony perforation. Similarly, large lesions can cause displacement and root resorption of adjacent teeth or elevation of the sinus floor (Figs. 41.1 and 41.2).

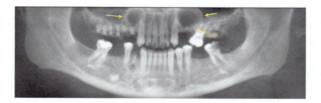

Fig. 41.1 Cone beam CT panoramic reconstruction showing multiple well-defined, periapical radiolucencies associated with carious teeth in the maxilla (yellow arrows). Cortication and peripheral sclerosis are noted. Tooth displacement is seen (orange arrow)

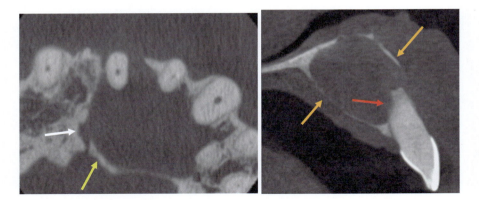

Fig. 41.2 CBCT axial and sagittal sections of a case of radicular cyst showing a well-defined, corticated, unilocular periapical radiolucent lesion centered around maxillary left central incisor (yellow arrow). Note the expansion and thinning of the cortical borders (orange arrows), loss of lamina dura (red arrow), and involvement of the nasopalatine canal (white arrow). (Courtesy to W. Alghamdi, BDS)

41.4 Histopathologic Features

The histopathologic features of all three types of inflammatory cysts are similar. The cyst is lined by stratified squamous epithelium that may demonstrate exocytosis, spongiosis, or hyperplasia. Occasionally this cyst may be lined by pseudostratified ciliated columnar epithelium or respiratory type of epithelium. The lining epithelium is of varying thickness from 6 to 20 cell layers with a great deal of proliferation and shows an arcading pattern with an intensely associated inflammatory process. Actual rete peg formation may sometimes be seen. The epithelium may be sometimes discontinuous and is frequently missing over the areas of intense inflammation. Occasionally, the lining epithelium may demonstrate a linear or arc-shaped calcification known as Rushton bodies or hyaline bodies. These linear or arc-shaped bodies are generally associated with the lining epithelium that appears amorphous in structure, eosinophilic in reaction, and brittle in nature. The etiology and pathogenesis of these bodies are not known. Rushton believed these bodies to be of odontogenic epithelial origin and probably a form of keratin. However, Sedano and Gorlin suggested that they might arise from thrombus formation in the small capillaries formed from the red blood cells.

The connective tissue wall of this cyst is composed of parallel bundles of collagen fibers that often appear compressed. Variable number of fibroblasts and small blood vessels are also present. A characteristic feature is the universal occurrence of the chronic inflammatory cells in the connective tissue immediately adjacent to the epithelium. In some cases, collections of cholesterol slits with associated multinucleated giant cells are found in the wall of the lesion. Dystrophic calcification may also be evident.

In the primary dentition, the radicular cysts reveal no change in their origin except for the rarity of cholesterol crystals. This may be explained by the fact that the lesions arising from the primary teeth exist for a shorter duration.

Occasionally, the wall of the inflammatory cyst will contain scattered hyaline bodies (pulse granuloma, giant cell hyaline angiopathy). These bodies appear as small circumscribed pools of eosinophilic material that exhibits a corrugated periphery of condensed collagen often surrounded by lymphocytes and multinucleated giant cells. The cystic lumen usually contains a fluid with low concentration of protein, occasionally a great deal of cholesterol, limited amounts of keratin, and cellular debris.

41.5   Differential Diagnosis

1. **Periapical rarefying osteitis:** Same etiological factors but smaller (<1 cm) in size with no cortication.
2. **Periapical osseous dysplasia:** Involved teeth are vital; occurs in the mandibular anterior region; multiple teeth involvement; and no cortication.
3. **Lateral periodontal cyst:** Can be easily confused with lateral periapical cyst. However, lamina dura and periodontal ligament space appear intact even though may be effaced.
4. **Other developmental odontogenic cysts in periapical location:** It is not uncommon to find cysts like odontogenic keratocyst in periapical location. In these cases, the involved teeth would be vital.

41.6   Treatment

When clinical and radiographic features point to a periapical inflammatory lesion, extraction or conservative nonsurgical endodontic therapy is performed. Larger lesions associated with teeth that can be restored have been treated successfully with conservative endodontic therapy and marsupialization, decompression, or fenestration.

Reference

1. Mass E, Kaplan I, Hirshberg A. A clinical and histopathological study of radicular cysts associated with primary molars. J Oral Pathol Med. 1995;24:458–61.

Cementoblastoma

42

Contents

42.1 Incidence... 185
42.2 Clinical Features.. 186
42.3 Radiographic Features.. 186
42.4 Differential Diagnosis.. 187
42.5 Histopathologic Features... 188
42.6 Treatment.. 188

Cementoblastoma is a benign neoplasm that forms a mass of cementum-like tissue. It resorbs and becomes fused to the root of a tooth.

Ulmansky et al. give credit to Norberg for being the first to recognize this tumor in 1930, but Bouquor and Lense credit Rodrguez who in 1930 called it as exostosis. Many authorities believe this neoplasm to represent the only true neoplasm of cementum.

42.1 Incidence

Regezi et al. found cementoblastoma to be <1% of their series of 706 odontogenic tumors, as did Daley et al. in Canada in their review of 403 odontogenic tumors. Jelic et al. found equal gender distribution in their study and a majority of the patients (66%) were aged between 15 and 30 years with the mandibular molar and premolar area commonly involved.

© The Author(s), under exclusive license to Springer Nature Singapore Pte Ltd. 2024
K. Paiwal et al., *Handbook of Oral and Maxillofacial Giant Cell Lesions*,
https://doi.org/10.1007/978-981-97-2863-3_42

42.2 Clinical Features

Cementoblastomas are rare neoplasms, representing <1% of all odontogenic tumors. The mandible (75%) is more commonly affected than the maxilla, with 90% arising in the molar and premolar region. Almost 50% involve the first permanent molar. Cementoblastomas rarely affect the deciduous dentition.

Children and young adults are the ones predominantly affected with about 50% under the age 20 and 75% below 30 years of age. Few studies report with no significant sex predilection, but others indicate a slight female predilection. The lesion causes jaw expansion and occasionally can cause gross bony swelling. Pain is a frequent complaint unlike other odontogenic tumors.

42.3 Radiographic Features

Cementoblastomas are mixed radiolucent-radiopaque lesions which are predominantly radiopaque and well-defined. The lesions have corticated borders, internal to which a well-defined radiolucent rim can be witnessed. The internal pattern may be uniformly radiopaque or resembling a wheel spoke pattern with radiating radiopaque lines arising from the center of the mass to the periphery (Fig. 42.1). The lesion is attached to the roots obscuring the root morphology. It may lead to external root resorption, although the vitality of the tooth is preserved. Larger lesions can cause bony expansion. In addition, cortical perforation may be observed in a few cases.

42.4 Differential Diagnosis

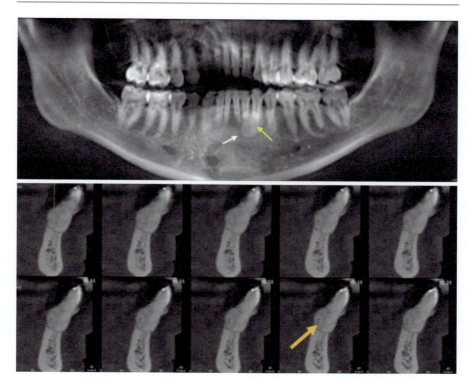

Fig. 42.1 CBCT panoramic reconstruction and cross-sectional view showing a well-defined, radiopaque lesion (yellow arrow) surrounded by a radiolucent rim (white arrow) attached to the roots of mandibular central incisors causing resorption of the roots (orange arrow) representing cementoblastoma. (Courtesy N. Shuff, DMD)

42.4 Differential Diagnosis

1. **Cemento-ossifying fibroma:** Concentric growth pattern, has thin, radiolucent rim (fibrous capsule), painless, not attached to the roots.
2. **Osteoid osteoma:** Painful, smaller in size with more sclerotic periphery.
3. **Osteoblastoma:** Less painful. This pain is not relieved by nonsteroidal anti-inflammatory medication. More aggressive with greater growth potential.
4. **Periapical osseous dysplasia:** Usually multifocal and painless. Mostly seen in the mandibular anterior region.
5. **Periapical sclerosing osteitis:** Associated with a non-vital tooth, loss of lamina dura, and widened periodontal ligament space.

42.5 Histopathologic Features

The relationship between the tooth root and the cementoblast-like cells indicates that it arises from the periodontal membrane. The histopathologic presentation of cementoblastoma closely resembles that of osteoblastoma with the primary distinguishing feature being tumor fusion with the involved tooth. It is characterized by the formation of sheets of cementum-like tissue, which may contain a large number of reversal lines and has a pagetoid appearance. Cells are enclosed within the hard tissue similar to osteocytes in the bone, while in the larger irregular spaces between the radiating trabeculae of calcified tissue and particularly around the periphery are many cementoblasts and cementoclasts. These cells are sometimes plump, pleomorphic, and hyperchromatic. It is believed that the process of tumor formation evolves in three stages: first is the osteolytic stage, followed by a cementoblastic stage and finally a mature inactive stage. At the periphery there are a broad unmineralized zone, an active growth area, and a mass of fibrous capsule. Cellular fibrovascular tissue is present between the mineralized trabeculae and multinucleated giant cells are often present.

42.6 Treatment

Benign cementoblastomas are surgically enucleated and rarely recur. Excision of the lesion and extraction of the associated tooth is the preferred treatment. Enucleation of the tumor by an apicoectomy after root canal treatment has been suggested.

Osteosarcoma

43

Contents

43.1	Etiology	190
43.2	Origin	190
43.3	Clinical Features	190
43.4	Oral Manifestations	190
43.5	Radiographic Features	191
43.6	Differential Diagnosis	193
43.7	Histopathologic Features	193
43.8	Diagnosis	194
43.9	Special Investigation	194
43.10	Treatment	194

Osteosarcoma is the malignancy of the mesenchymal cells that have the ability of producing osteoid or immature bone. It is the most common malignant tumor of bone with the exception of multiple myeloma.

The World Health Organization (WHO) recognizes several variants that differ in location, clinical behavior, and degree of cytologic atypia. The most commonly occurring is the conventional osteosarcoma constituting 20% of primary bone tumors, which arises centrally within the bone and can be divided into osteoblastic, fibroblastic, and chondroblastic variants depending upon the predominant cell type.

Other variants of osteosarcomas listed by WHO include intramedullary low-grade osteosarcoma, parosteal osteosarcoma, and telangiectatic, low-grade intraosseous, and small cell variants. In the simplest classification scheme, osteosarcomas can be divided into primary forms which arise de novo and secondary forms, which arise as a complication of a known underlying process, such as Paget's disease of bone or a history of radiation exposure. The majority of osteosarcomas demonstrate intramedullary origin, but a small number may be juxtacortical or rarely extra-skeletal.

© The Author(s), under exclusive license to Springer Nature Singapore Pte Ltd. 2024
K. Paiwal et al., *Handbook of Oral and Maxillofacial Giant Cell Lesions*,
https://doi.org/10.1007/978-981-97-2863-3_43

43.1 Etiology

The cause of osteosarcoma is unknown, but genetic mutations appear to be important in their pathogenesis. Mutation in TP53 tumor suppressor gene and overexpression of MDM2 gene, which binds to and inactivates TP53 gene product and an expression difference in C-erb-B2 gene, is noted. Germ line mutations of RB (retinoblastoma) gene predispose to the development of osteosarcoma and retinoblastoma. It also occurs as a complication of Paget's disease or following a history of radiation exposure or as a postirradiation complication in patients treated for fibrous dysplasia.

43.2 Origin

From a biologic perspective, the cells of origin are by no means well-defined, and it is likely that they are not osteoblasts, but undifferentiated mesenchymal precursors with osteogenic potential. Cellular heterogeneity exists within the tumor with fibroblasts, chondroblasts, and osteoblasts sharing a common lineage.

43.3 Clinical Features

Extragnathic osteosarcomas demonstrate a bimodal age distribution. Most arise in patients between the ages of 10 and 20 years, with few diagnosed in adults over the age of 50 years. Most of these tumors occur in the distal femoral and proximal tibial metaphysis. In older patients, the axial bones and flat bones can also be involved.

Osteosarcomas present as progressively enlarging tumors often painful masses that may come to attention because of the fracture of the involved bone. A definite history of trauma preceding the development or at least the discovery of the tumor is noticed in approximately half of the reported cases. Conventional osteosarcomas are aggressive lesions and metastasis through blood in their early course. The lung is the main organ of metastases. Secondary osteosarcomas occur in the older age group. They commonly develop as a complication of Paget's disease or a previous radiation exposure or rarely in patients with fibrous dysplasia.

43.4 Oral Manifestations

Osteosarcoma of the jaws is a rare aggressive malignancy constituting 5–13% of all cases of skeletal osteosarcomas. These gnathic tumors generally occur in the third and fourth decade of life but have also been reported to occur in young children. The mean age for patients with osteosarcoma of the jaw is about 33 years, which is 10–15 years older than the mean age for osteosarcomas of the long bones. Males are more commonly affected than females.

The mandible is frequently affected than the maxilla. Mandibular tumors arise more frequently in the posterior body and horizontal ramus rather than the ascending ramus. Maxillary lesions are discovered more commonly in the inferior portion (alveolar ridge, sinus floor, palate) than the superior aspects (zygoma, orbital rim).

Swelling and pain are the most common symptoms. Paresthesia of one of the branches of the trigeminal nerve is an additional finding in osteosarcomas of the jaw. The swelling in the facial region can be detected at an early stage. Maxillary tumors may extend into the sinus. Loosening of teeth, paresthesia, and nasal obstruction may also be noted.

Osteosarcomas spread microscopically along the bone marrow spaces, mandibular canal, the periodontal ligament space, the mental nerve, and the inferior alveolar nerve.

43.5 Radiographic Features

The radiographic findings vary from dense sclerosis to a mixed sclerotic and radiolucent lesion to an entirely radiolucent process.

The peripheral border of the lesion is usually ill-defined and indistinct, making it difficult to determine the extent of the tumor radiographically. The lesions cause destruction of the cortical borders including mandibular canal, antrum of the nasal cavity. If the cortical borders are destroyed, a soft tissue mass emanating from the bone may be observed. If the periosteum is elevated, radiating radiopaque lines may be seen arising from the surface of the bone to the exterior, giving a "sunburst" or "hair-on-end" appearance. In a few cases, especially in the long bone, a triangular radiopacity may be seen near the edges of the bone where the cortical borders are breached, known as Codman triangle. If the periodontal space of the adjacent teeth is invaded, there will be irregular widening, referred to as the Garrington sign. Occasionally, there might be resorption of the roots of the teeth involved and this is described as "spiking" resorption due to the tapered narrow root (Figs. 43.1, 43.2, 43.3, and 43.4).

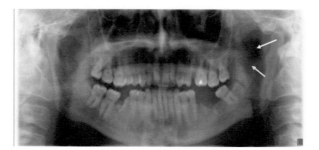

Fig. 43.1 Panoramic radiograph of a case of osteosarcoma showing radiating radiopaque lines arising from the left maxillary tuberosity superimposed over the coronoid process (yellow arrow). A radiopaque entity is also noted superior to the left sigmoid notch (white arrow)

Fig. 43.2 MDCT axial image of the same patient showing a soft tissue mass occupying the entire left maxillary sinus (yellow arrow) causing destruction of the medial and posterolateral walls, extending into the nasal cavity (white arrow). Faint radiopaque striae are seen within the soft tissue mass (orange arrows)

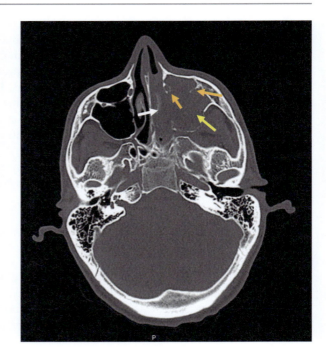

Fig. 43.3 Contrast enhanced MDCT axial image of the same patient at the level of parapharyngeal space showing a well-defined, hypodense lesion with minimal enhancement on the left side (yellow arrow) involving the lateral pterygoid muscle and displacing the airway to the contralateral side. A small, calcified area is seen within the entity (white arrow)

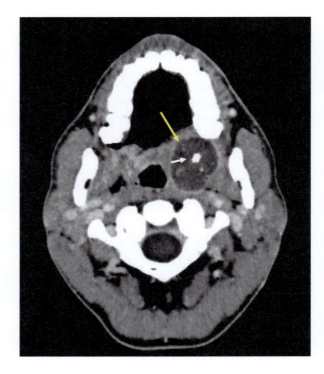

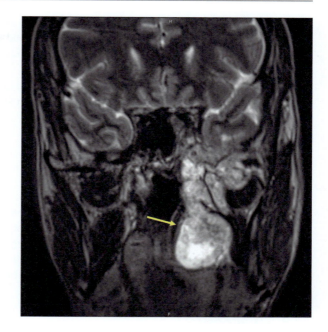

Fig. 43.4 Contrast enhanced T2 weighted MRI coronal image of the same patient showing a hyperintense enhancing lesion on the left side extending from the parapharyngeal space to the base of the skull (yellow arrow)

43.6 Differential Diagnosis

1. **Chondrosarcoma:** Less common, radiolucent nidus present within the lesion, more common in the anterior jaw, and coronoid and condylar processes.
2. **Osteomyelitis:** Clinical signs of infection usually present, less bone destruction, mostly with sequestrum formation and periosteal reaction (onion skin pattern).
3. **Osteoid osteoma:** Painful and less destructive behavior.
4. **Osteoblastoma:** Less painful and this pain is not relieved by nonsteroidal anti-inflammatory medication; less destructive behavior.
5. **Fibrous dysplasia:** Expansion is more regular with no periosteal reaction and less destructive behavior.
6. **Metastasis:** Clinical history reveals primary lesion and less sclerotic pattern.

43.7 Histopathologic Features

Osteosarcomas originate from bone cells and this can produce a highly pleomorphic picture in which bone formation does not necessarily predominate. The tumor cells are variable in shape and size; many are large and hyperchromatic, with prominent mitotic figures, particularly in highly cellular areas. Cells resembling osteoblasts, chondroblasts, and fibroblasts can be seen; giant cells may be conspicuous, but many are of indeterminate appearance. These giant cells are often seen in osteosarcomas arising as a complication due to radiation.

The amount of matrix produced in the tumor may vary considerably. In some instances, osteoid production may be very minimal and difficult to demonstrate. Most osteosarcomas of the jaws tend to be better differentiated than osteosarcomas of the extragnathic skeleton.

Depending on the relative amounts of osteoid, cartilage, or collagen fibers produced by the tumor, many pathologists classify osteosarcomas into the following types:

1. Osteoblastic osteosarcoma
2. Chondroblastic osteosarcoma
3. Fibroblastic osteosarcoma

Microscopically, low-grade intraosseous osteosarcoma is essentially a spindle-cell tumor with irregular bone production, low cellularity, fewer than 4 mitoses per 10 high-power fields, and an absence of pronounced atypia. Heavy seams of osteoid embedded in a collagenous stroma may be seen, or an abundant osteoid with osteoblastic rimming may mimic osteoblastic fibroma or a fibromyxoid change.

43.8 Diagnosis

The diagnosis depends upon the type of biopsy. While et al. reported fine needle aspiration gives 80% accuracy in the diagnosis of osteosarcomas. Serum alkaline phosphatase levels may be raised in cases where new bone formation predominates.

43.9 Special Investigation

Osteoclastin, a bone-specific protein, is useful in distinguishing osteosarcomas from malignant fibrous histiocytoma. Alkaline phosphatase activity in the imprint preparation before fixation is considered diagnosis along with radiographs.

43.10 Treatment

Early radical excision of osteosarcomas of the jaws is the first requirement. This involves maxillectomy or mandibulectomy with excision of any soft tissue extension of the tumor. Excision may be combined with pre- as well as postoperative radiotherapy and adjuvant chemotherapy. With radical surgery, the 5-year survival rate has been reported to be up to 80%.

The prognosis depends mainly on the extent of tumor, the site of tumor, and metastasis of the tumor. The tumor rarely metastasizes to the lungs and the overall incidence has been found to be not higher than 18%. Metastasis to the regional lymph nodes is found in <10% of the cases.

Actinomycosis

44

Contents

44.1	Oral Lesions	197
44.2	Laboratory Diagnosis	197
44.3	Culture	198
44.4	Histological Features	198
44.5	Treatment	198
References		198

Actinomycosis is a chronic granulomatous, suppurative, and fibrosing disease caused by anaerobic, gram-positive, non-acid-fast, branched, filamentous bacteria. The most commonly isolated organism is *Actinomyces israelii*, although *A. naeslundii*, *A. viscosus*, *A. odontolyticus*, and *A. propionica* have also been shown to cause the human disease.

It was first described in the early nineteenth century as a disease entity found in cattle. In 1826 LeBlanc had observed actinomycotic tumors in cattle and described them erroneously as osteosarcomas. Langenbeck in 1845 was probably the first to describe the disease in humans but his work was not published until 40 years later. The first published clinical description of the entity was by Lebet in 1857.

Actinomycetes are traditionally considered to be transitional forms between bacteria and fungi. Like fungi they form a mycelia network of branching filaments, but, unlike bacteria, they are thin, possess cell walls containing muramic acid, have prokaryotic nuclei, and are susceptible to antibacterial antibiotics. They are therefore true bacteria, bearing a superficial resemblance to fungi. They are gram- positive, non-motile, non-sporing, non-capsulated filaments that break up into bacillary and coccoid elements.

Bollinger [1] found mold-like organisms in the lesion of "lumpy jaw" (actinomycosis) in cattle. Harz coined the name actinomyces to refer to the ray-like appearance of the organisms in the granules that characterize the lesions (actinomyces, meaning ray fungus).

© The Author(s), under exclusive license to Springer Nature Singapore Pte Ltd. 2024
K. Paiwal et al., *Handbook of Oral and Maxillofacial Giant Cell Lesions*,
https://doi.org/10.1007/978-981-97-2863-3_44

Wolff and Israel [2] isolated an anaerobic bacillus from human lesions and produced experimental infection in rabbits and guinea pigs. This was named *Actinomyces israelii* and causes human actinomycosis. Actinomycosis in cattle is produced by *A. bovis*.

The word actinomycosis is a Greek derivative that combines aktino, which refers to the radiating appearance of the sulfur granules, and mykos, which labels this condition as a mycotic disease.

Actinomycosis is a rare disease reported worldwide and is common in the rural areas and among agricultural workers. The incidence of the infection has been greatly reduced due to the widespread use of antibiotics; it is commonly seen in young healthy adults and 80% of the cases appear in patients over the age of 29 years. Benhoff had noted a special incidence in the middle cycles (fourth to sixth decades).

The infection in humans is usually endogenous in origin. These organisms are present as commensals in the oral cavity, alimentary tract, and vagina. The organisms may invade, through trauma, foreign objects, or poor oral hygiene. Actinomycosis is characterized by the development of indurate swellings mainly in the connective tissue with suppuration and discharge of sulfur granules. The lesion often points toward the skin, leading to multiple sinuses.

Actinomycosis occurs in humans in four main clinical forms:

1. Cervicofacial actinomycosis
2. Thoracic actinomycosis
3. Abdominal actinomycosis
4. Pelvic actinomycosis

1. **Cervicofacial Actinomycosis**

This is the commonest form of actinomycosis (40–60%) infection with indurated lesions on the cheek and the submaxillary regions and has the best prognosis. The portal of entry is usually through a disruption of the mucosal barrier after trauma or dental manipulations, and it requires an oxidoreductive condition provided by a particular bacterial ecosystem. The other possible routes of entry are tonsils, carious teeth, periodontal disease, or trauma following tooth extraction. Initially, the lesion develops as a firm swelling in the lower jaw (lumpy jaw). The organisms may remain localized in the subjacent soft tissues or spread to involve the salivary glands and bone or skin of the face and neck. With time the mass breaks down and abscesses occur, discharging pus containing tiny yellow sulfur granules. The skin overlying the abscess is purplish red and indurated or often fluctuant. It is common for the sinus to heal, but because of the chronicity of the disease, new abscesses may develop and perforate the skin surface. Thus, the patient over a period of time may show a great deal of scarring and disfigurement of the skin.

The infection may extend deep to involve the maxilla or mandible and cause extensive destruction. Bone marrow involvement can lead to rapid extension of the process, which can ultimately result in cranial, cervical, vertebral, and central nervous system dissemination. Focal CNS infection occurs when access is gained to the meningitis, meningoencephalitis, and brain abscess. The signs and symptoms depend upon the location of the abscess and include focal neurological findings as well as signs of increased intracranial pressure.

2. **Thoracic Actinomycosis**

This manifests as lesions in the lung that may involve the pleura and pericardium which spread outward through the chest wall. Aspiration of the organism from the oral cavity may cause infection in the lungs or extension of infection from abdominal or hepatic lesions. Initially the disease resembles pneumonia but subsequently spreads to the whole of the lung, pleura, ribs, as well as vertebrae with generalized signs and symptoms of fever as well as chills accompanied by a productive cough and pleural pain.

3. **Abdominal Actinomycosis**

The lesions occur usually around the cecum, with involvement of the neighboring tissues and abdominal wall. Sometimes the infection spreads to the liver via the portal vein. It is an extremely serious form of the disease and carries a high mortality rate. The abdominal infection results from swallowing of organisms from the oral cavity or extension from thoracic cavity. In addition to generalized signs and symptoms of fever, chills, nausea, and vomiting, intestinal manifestations develop.

4. **Pelvic Actinomycosis**

Infection in the pelvis occurs as a complication of intrauterine contraceptive devices (IUCDs).

44.1   Oral Lesions

Actinomyces have been incriminated in inflammatory diseases of the gums (gingivitis and periodontitis) and with sublingual plaques leading to root surface caries.

44.2   Laboratory Diagnosis

The diagnosis is made by demonstrating actinomycetes in the lesion by microscopy and by isolation in culture. The specimen to be collected is pus. In pulmonary disease, sputum is collected.

Sulfur granules may be demonstrated in the pus by shaking it up in a test tube with some saline. On standing, the granule sediment may be withdrawn by a capillary pipette. Granules may also be obtained by applying gauze pads over the discharging sinus.

The granules are white or yellowish and range in size from minute specks to about 5 mm. They are crushed between slides, stained by Gram stain, and examined microscopically. The granules are bacterial colonies and will be found to consist of a dense network of thin gram-positive filaments, surrounded by a peripheral zone of swollen radiating club-shaped structures, presenting a sunray appearance. The clubs are believed to be antigen-antibody complexes.

44.3 Culture

When organisms are washed and inoculated into thioglycolate liquid medium or streaked on heart brain infusion agar and incubated anaerobically at 37 °C, *A. bovis* produces general turbidity, whereas *A. Israelii* produces small "spidery colonies" in 48–72 h that become heaped up, white, and irregular or smooth, large colonies in 10 days. The isolate is identified by microscopy biochemical reactions and fluorescent antibody methods.

44.4 Histological Features

The typical lesion of actinomycosis, either in soft tissue or bone, is essentially a granulomatous reaction with central caseous necrosis within which may be characteristic colonies of microorganisms. These colonies appear to be floating in the sea of polymorphonuclear around the periphery of the lesion. The individual colony, which may appear round or lobulated and is made up of mesh work of filaments that stain with hematoxylin, shows eosinophilia of the peripheral club-shaped ends of the filaments, representative of secreted immunoglobulins. This peculiar arrangement of radiating filaments is the basis for use of the term "ray fungus." The center of each abscess contains the bacterial colony, "sulfur granules" characterized by radiating filaments (hence previously known as ray fungus) with hyaline, eosinophilic, club-like ends.

44.5 Treatment

Treatment is centered on surgical manipulations and high-dose long-term antibiotics as the antibiotics have to penetrate the hypovascular tissue with low oxidation-reduction potential. Maxillary sinus involvement can be treated by Caldwell-Luc approach and sphenoidectomy for the sphenoid sinus. Bone involvement must be treated by curettage and ablation sequestra are necessary. Uncomplicated cases should initially be treated with IV penicillin G at doses of 3–12 million units daily until the lesions have subsided. Patients with more severe infection, like osteomyelitis, are treated with IV penicillin G at doses of 12–20 million units per day in four equal doses.

Other antibiotics that can be used when patients are allergic to penicillin include erythromycin, tetracycline, clindamycin, rifampicin, and chloramphenicol; due to the fibrotic and avascular nature of the tumor, some authors suggest the use of hyperbaric oxygen.

References

1. https://scholar.google.com/scholar_lookup?author=Bollinger+O.&publication_year=1877&title=Ueber+eine+neue+Pilzkrankheit+beim+Rinde&journal=Zentralblatt+Medizinische+Wissenschaft.
2. https://ia600708.us.archive.org/view_archive.php?archive=/22/items/crossref-pre-1909-scholarlyworks/10.1007%252Fbf01936281.zip&file=10.1007%252Fbf01937693.pdf.

Cat Scratch Disease

45

Contents

45.1	Epidemiology and Transmission	199
45.2	Mode of Spread	200
45.3	Clinical Features	200
45.4	Mild Systemic Symptoms Associated with Typical Cat Scratch Disease	200
45.5	Atypical Clinical Manifestation of Cat Scratch Disease	200
45.6	Histopathology	201
45.7	Diagnosis and Management	201
45.8	Treatment	201
Reference		201

Cat scratch disease is a self-limiting lymphadenitis caused by *Bartonella henselae*. The disease begins in the skin but classically spreads to the adjacent lymph nodes. Cat scratch disease is considered one of the most common causes of chronic (greater than 3-week duration) regional lymphadenopathy in children and adolescents. It is primarily a disease of childhood, with 90% of patients younger than 18 years.

The first case was reported by Debre et al. [1]. Earlier it was believed to be viral in origin but in 1988 isolation and culture of the organism were achieved. The causative organism was initially named *Rochalimaea henselae* but was reclassified as *Bartonella henselae*.

45.1 Epidemiology and Transmission

Reports indicate that CSD is seasonal, with peaks of the disease occurring in the fall and winter months in temperate climates and extending to July and August in warmer climates. Cat scratch disease occurs worldwide and all ethnic groups are affected. Males appear to contract the disease more often than do females and the affected families have at least one cat and most often kittens.

© The Author(s), under exclusive license to Springer Nature Singapore Pte Ltd. 2024
K. Paiwal et al., *Handbook of Oral and Maxillofacial Giant Cell Lesions*,
https://doi.org/10.1007/978-981-97-2863-3_45

Transmission of CSD occurs from a bite, scratch, or petting, as a result of direct contact with the cat's saliva. The saliva is deposited on an infected cat's fur and claws from self-grooming.

45.2 Mode of Spread

The organism typically enters the skin through a scratch, bite, or a previous site of injury. Almost all cases arise after contact with a cat, usually a kitten. On rare occasions, dogs and monkeys have served as the vector or it is also seen uncommonly after a splinter or thorn injury.

45.3 Clinical Features

The inoculation papule progresses through a series of stages: changing from a papule to an opaque, fluid-filled vesicle, then to a crusty, maculopapular lesion, and, finally, to a macule which may last several months. As children often hold kittens close to their chest and face, most inoculation lesions occur on the upper body, with approximately 80% of enlarged nodes found on the head, neck, and axilla. This takes the form of regional lymphadenopathy, most frequently in the axilla and neck 2 weeks after the scratch, and may be accompanied in early stages with a low-grade fever, chills, malaise, or even abdominal pain. A positive history of contact with cats and regional lymphadenopathy involving single or multiple nodes proximal to an inoculation site is a fair diagnosis of CSD. Although most CSD patients have single node involvement, lymphadenopathy may occur in more than one site.

The lymph nodes gradually become soft and fluctuant owing to necrosis and suppuration. Occasionally an abscessed lymph node will perforate skin and drain. The lymph node enlargement may regress over the next 2–4 months in some patients. Rarely, patients develop encephalitis, osteomyelitis, or thrombocytopenia.

45.4 Mild Systemic Symptoms Associated with Typical Cat Scratch Disease

These include fatigue, headache, abdominal pain, splenomegaly, myalgias, low-grade fever, exanthema, malaise, pharyngitis, nausea, and vomiting.

45.5 Atypical Clinical Manifestation of Cat Scratch Disease

These include parinaud's oculoglandular syndrome, osteolytic bone lesions, bacillary angiomatosis, central nervous system involvement, erythema nodosum, brain abscess, bacillary hepatitis, and splenitis.

Parinaud's oculoglandular syndrome is characterized by an ocular granuloma and conjunctivitis associated with swelling of the parotid gland secondary to preauricular and/or submandibular lymphadenopathy. Conjunctival lesions are self-limiting and resolve after several weeks.

45.6 Histopathology

Initially, sarcoids like granulomas are formed that develop central necrosis with accumulation of neutrophils. Epithelioid cells and multinucleated giant cells are occasionally seen. The microbe is extracellular and can be visualized only by silver stains or electron microscopy. Diagnosis is based on a history of exposure to cats, clinical findings, positive skin test to the microbial antigen, and distinctive changes in the lymph nodes.

45.7 Diagnosis and Management

Most cases of CSD are diagnosed by the following criteria: (a) history of kitten/cat contact with evidence of scratches or bites, (b) inoculation lesions, (c) regional lymphadenitis, and (d) a positive serum IFA or EIA test.

Although the CSD skin test has a high degree of specificity, the test is not standardized, is not available commercially, and is no longer recommended. Currently available for diagnosis purposes are the serum immunofluorescent-antibody (IFA) test for *B. henselae*, which has 91% positive value, 96% specificity, and 84% sensitivity, and the enzyme immunoassay (EIA) test, which is thought to be the most accurate.

45.8 Treatment

Treatment for uncomplicated CSD remains controversial, and the literature review reveals differing opinions regarding the use of antibiotics relative to their efficacy, appropriate dosage, and duration of therapy. Generally, CSD is a self-limiting condition with regional lymphadenopathy that spontaneously resolves in approximately 2–4 months with no treatment. Oral rifampicin is found to be more effective; ciprofloxacin and intramuscular gentamicin were prescribed for severely ill patients. Incision and drainage of the involved lymph node may be necessary.

Reference

1. https://pubmed.ncbi.nlm.nih.gov/9203735/.

Blastomycosis

46

Contents

46.1 Epidemiology.. 203
46.2 Morphology... 204
46.3 Mode of Infection.. 204
46.4 Clinical Features... 204
46.5 Oral Manifestations.. 205
46.6 Laboratory Findings.. 205
46.7 Culture... 205
46.8 Histologic Findings.. 205
46.9 Treatment.. 206

It is a granulomatous fungal infection caused by *Blastomyces dermatitidis*, a thermally dimorphic fungus that initiates disease by infecting the lungs. It is characterized by the formation of suppurative and granulomatous lesion in any part of the body but with a marked predilection for the lungs and skin.

The term blastomycosis has sometimes been taken to include a range of granulomatous systemic mycosis, including South American blastomycosis, North American blastomycosis, coccidioidomycosis, and cryptococcosis, but is now generally retracted to North and South American forms. In 1894, Gilchrist first described it in the United States.

46.1 Epidemiology

Blastomycosis appears to be endemic in Southern Canada, Central Midwest, and Southeast and Atlantic coastal states of the United States. As the infection is more confined to the North American continent, it is known as "North American

© The Author(s), under exclusive license to Springer Nature Singapore Pte Ltd. 2024
K. Paiwal et al., *Handbook of Oral and Maxillofacial Giant Cell Lesions*,
https://doi.org/10.1007/978-981-97-2863-3_46

blastomycosis." It may serve as an indicator of human disease because of the shared environment. Blastomycosis is reported in other animals, including the horse, cow, cat, bat, and lion.

46.2 Morphology

In tissue and in culture at 37 °C, the fungus appears as budding yeast cells, which are large (7–20 μm) and spherical, with thick, double-contoured walls. Each cell contains only a single broad-based bud.

46.3 Mode of Infection

The infection occurs by inhalation of aerosolized conidial forms of the fungus from its natural soil habitat. Once inhaled into the lungs, the conidia transform at body temperature to the yeast phase (thermal dimorphism). Then, they multiply and may disseminate through the blood and lymphatics to other organs. The evoked granulomatous inflammatory response has an initial influx of neutrophils, followed by macrophage resulting in granuloma formation.

46.4 Clinical Features

Blastomycosis was thought to occur more often in males than females; however, recent reports do not indicate a significant sex difference. The outdoor workers are affected commonly. The mean age at diagnosis is approximately 45 years. Most patients are aged 30–69 years; however, persons of any age can acquire the disease. Blastomycosis generally takes two forms: pulmonary with dissemination and chronic cutaneous disease.

Acute blastomycosis presents with prodromal symptoms such as a flu-like illness with fever, chills, myalgia, headache, nonproductive cough (which resolves within days), or a productive cough and pleuritic chest pain. The sputum is mucopurulent or purulent. Hemoptysis may be present that resembles tuberculosis or malignancy. Pulmonary lesions may disseminate and involve the skin.

Chronic blastomycosis is more common than acute forms and it may mimic tuberculosis commonly manifesting as pulmonary infection. It may be asymptomatic in nearly 50% of the patients. In others, the median incubation period, from inhalation of the fungus to manifestation of symptoms, is 45 days (range 21–106 days). Pulmonary symptoms of varying severity are common and most often occur without any symptoms of dissemination to other organs. Extrapulmonary dissemination more often occurs in patients with chronic pulmonary illness and in those who are immunocompromised.

The skin is the commonest site of extrapulmonary blastomycosis and is involved in about 20–40% of the cases. Skin lesions are more common on the face, neck, and extremities. Lesions begin as papules, pustules, or subcutaneous nodules. Within a few weeks to months, the primary lesions evolve into ulcers, with indurated dusky or violaceous granulomatous or verrucous borders, or into vegetating plaques. Typically, the border is arciform, contains numerous tiny pustules or microabscesses covered with crust, and rises abruptly from the normal surrounding skin. Over a period of months to years, the lesions enlarge, eventually involving a substantial portion of the face, and produce severe disfigurement. As the lesions enlarge, they heal centrally, with atrophic scar studded with telangiectasia. The skin lesions are described as "chancriform" and are accompanied by nodular lymphangitis.

46.5 Oral Manifestations

The extensions of cutaneous infection may involve the lips or disseminated blastomycosis may produce ulcerative lesions affecting the oral mucosa. Other areas affected in order of frequency are the bones (10–25%), prostate and other genitourinary organs (5–15%), and the meninges and brain (5%). In rare instances, any organ can be affected, including the breast, eye, larynx, trachea, and ear. Reactivation of blastomycosis may occur after a pulmonary infection that has resolved with or without treatment. Extrapulmonary site is rarely a site of reactivation (e.g., skin, bone, brain).

46.6 Laboratory Findings

Sputum Examination: Place a small sample of freshly expectorated sputum on a slide and digest it with drops of potassium hydroxide. Cover it with a coverslip and examine it under the microscope. Yeasts, 8–20 μm in size, with single, broad-based buds, double refractile walls, and multiple nuclei are extremely characteristics of *B. dermatitidis*.

46.7 Culture

Specimens can also be cultured on Sabouraud's and enriched media such as brain-heart infusion.

An enzyme immunoassay (EIA) for antibodies to the A antigen of *B. dermatitidis* is a more sensitive test and titers greater than 1:32 strongly support the diagnosis.

46.8 Histologic Findings

The yeast forms are best visualized with a periodic acid-Schiff (PAS) stain. The methenamine silver and Papanicolaou are other reliable stains. Skin lesions of disseminated blastomycosis are characterized by pseudoepitheliomatous hyperplasia of the epidermis, intraepidermal microabscesses, and a suppurating granulomatous reaction in the dermis.

The hyperplastic epidermis lacks the cytologic atypia of squamous cell carcinoma and such skin lesions are also called pseudoepitheliomatous (pseudocarcinomatous) hyperplasia. Intraepidermal abscesses contain abundant neutrophils and organisms. The organisms are best visualized with the diastase-digested PAS staining procedure or with the methenamine silver stain. Yeasts are present extracellularly in the dermis or intracellularly in multinucleated giant cells. Intracellular yeasts are easily identified on routine hematoxylin and eosin-stained sections of skin as punched-out "holes" in cytoplasm of the giant cells. The inflammatory infiltrate is polymorphous, containing lymphocytes, histiocytes, and neutrophils. Tuberculoid granuloma formation is unusual, but if it occurs, it is not accompanied by caseation.

46.9 Treatment

Amphotericin B is highly effective and is the drug of choice in overwhelming or life-threatening blastomycosis (e.g., ARDS, CNS involvement, immunocompromised patients). However, it is associated with several toxic effects, most notably renal impairment. Itraconazole is the drug of choice in mild-to-moderate pulmonary and extrapulmonary blastomycosis without CNS involvement. In severe cases amphotericin B is advised as a cumulative dose of 1G followed by itraconazole for 2–4 months.

Rhinosporidiosis

47

Contents

47.1   Mode of Infection... 207
47.2   Clinical Features... 207
47.3   Oral Manifestations... 208
47.4   Diagnosis... 208
      47.4.1   Smears... 208
47.5   Histopathology.. 208
47.6   Treatment... 208
Reference.. 208

Rhinosporidiosis is a chronic granulomatous disease caused by fungus *Rhinosporidium seeberi* and is characterized by the development of polyps in the nose, mouth, and eye but rarely in the genitalia or in other mucous membranes.

47.1   Mode of Infection

The mode of infection is not known. Rhinosporidiosis was first identified in Argentina but the large majority of cases come from India and Sri Lanka.

47.2   Clinical Features

The initial symptoms include nasal irritation accompanied by a mucoid discharge. Lesions develop as small, sessile, papillomatous lesions, which eventually enlarge, become pedunculated, and protrude from the nares. These appear soft and friable and are highly vascular. The mucosal surfaces, conjunctiva, mouth, larynx, bronchus, or anus may also be involved but vagina or skin is rarely affected.

© The Author(s), under exclusive license to Springer Nature Singapore Pte
Ltd. 2024
K. Paiwal et al., *Handbook of Oral and Maxillofacial Giant Cell Lesions*,
https://doi.org/10.1007/978-981-97-2863-3_47

47.3 Oral Manifestations

The oronasopharyngeal lesions are often accompanied by a mucoid discharge and appear as soft, red, polypoid tumor-like growth, which may spread to the pharynx and larynx. The lesions are vascular and bleed readily.

The oral lesions have been reviewed by Prabhu et al. [1] and they cited that any intraoral site may be involved in rhinosporidiosis and soft palate appears to be the most frequent site of oral involvement.

47.4 Diagnosis

47.4.1 Smears

An impression smear from the lesion or secretions mixed with a drop of water and examined under the microscope will reveal sporangia and spores. The causative fungus *Rhinosporidium seeberi* has not been cultivated. Histopathological diagnosis of the lesions is of great diagnostic importance.

47.5 Histopathology

The lesion is composed of a large number of fungal spherules embedded in a stroma of connective tissue and capillaries. The organisms appear as sporangia containing large numbers of round or ovoid endospores. The surrounding tissue reaction itself is a nonspecific one consisting of vascular granulation tissue with focal abscess formation and occasional multinucleated giant cells.

47.6 Treatment

Surgical removal of the growth and application of cautery is the treatment recommended.

Reference

1. Prabhu SR, Wilson DF, Daftary DK, Johnson NW. Oral diseases in the tropics. 1st ed. Oxford university press. Delhi. 1993.

Giant Cell Arteritis (Temporal Arteritis)

48

Contents

48.1	Clinical Features	209
48.2	Pathogenesis	210
48.3	Histopathologic Features	210
48.4	Diagnosis	210
48.5	Treatment	210

Giant cell temporal arteritis, the most common of the vasculitis, is an acute and chronic, often granulomatous, inflammation of the arteries of large to small size. It affects principally the temporal arteries but also the vertebral and ophthalmic arteries. Its cause remains unknown, but autoimmunity to the elastic lamina of the artery has been proposed.

48.1 Clinical Features

Temporal arteritis occurs most frequently in older people and is rare before the age of 50 years. Symptoms are vague and constitutional: fever, fatigue, weight loss without localizing signs, and symptoms such as facial pain or headache, often intense along the course of the superficial artery which may be painful to palpation. It affects women more frequently than men.

The superficial temporal artery eventually appears erythematous, swollen, tortuous, or rarely bilateral. Since the mandibular and lingual arteries may be involved, a throbbing pain in the jaw or tongue may be an early sign or even a presenting sign. A serious complication in untreated patients is the ischemia of the eye, which may lead to progressive loss of vision or sudden blindness. These visual manifestations may be prevented by early diagnosis and prompt therapy. Patients with polymyalgia rheumatica will have accompanying joint and muscle pain.

© The Author(s), under exclusive license to Springer Nature Singapore Pte Ltd. 2024
K. Paiwal et al., *Handbook of Oral and Maxillofacial Giant Cell Lesions*,
https://doi.org/10.1007/978-981-97-2863-3_48

48.2 Pathogenesis

The cause remains relatively elusive. However, much evidence points to a T-cell-mediated immune response to an unknown possible vessel wall antigen with the presence of CD4+ T cells in the lesions, an association with certain HLA-DR antigens, and the presence of a clonal T-cell population at multiple affected sites suggesting a response to specific antigen.

48.3 Histopathologic Features

The disease is characterized by granulomatous inflammation of the inner half of the media centered on the internal elastic membrane with narrowing of the lumen from edema and proliferation of the intima. Necrosis of the smooth muscle and elastic lamina is frequent. A variable number of foreign body-type multinucleated giant cells are mixed with macrophages, plasma cells, and lymphocytes. Both CD4+ and CD8+ lymphocytes are found. Thrombosis or complete occlusion of the lumen is not unusual.

48.4 Diagnosis

Laboratory abnormalities include an elevated erythrocyte sedimentation rate (ESR) and anemia. Abnormal C-reactive protein may also be an important early finding.

48.5 Treatment

Temporal arteritis responds well to systemic steroids and local corticosteroids; the symptoms subside within a few days. Permanent loss of vision occurs in more than 50% of untreated patients and even in occasional refractory patients. With some cases, the vascular involvement is so widespread that the disease is fatal, even with corticosteroid therapy.

Pyogenic Granuloma

49

Contents

49.1 Etiology.. 211
49.2 Clinical Features... 212

The pyogenic granuloma is a distinctive clinical entity originating as a response to a nonspecific infection. It is a common tumor-like growth of the oral cavity that is considered to be nonneoplastic in nature. Although it was originally thought to be caused by pyogenic organisms, it is now believed to be unrelated to infection. In spite of its name, it is not a true granuloma.

49.1 Etiology

Pyogenic granuloma was originally thought to be a botryomycosis infection, an infection in horses thought to be transmissible to man. Subsequent studies suggested that the lesion was due to infection by either staphylococci or streptococci. It is now generally agreed that pyogenic granuloma arises as a result of some minor trauma to the tissues, which provide a pathway for the invasion of nonspecific types of microorganisms. The tissues respond in a characteristic manner to these organisms of low virulence by proliferation of a vascular type of connective tissue.

It is also thought to represent an exuberant tissue response to local irritation or trauma. Local factors such as calculus, food debris, and overhanging margins of dental restorations are important irritants.

© The Author(s), under exclusive license to Springer Nature Singapore Pte Ltd. 2024
K. Paiwal et al., *Handbook of Oral and Maxillofacial Giant Cell Lesions*,
https://doi.org/10.1007/978-981-97-2863-3_49

49.2 Clinical Features

The pyogenic granuloma of the oral cavity arises most frequently on the gingiva but may also be found on the lips, tongue, and buccal mucosa and occasionally in other areas.

The pyogenic granuloma is a smooth or lobulated mass that is usually pedunculated or sessile. The surface is characteristically ulcerated and shows a tendency for hemorrhage either spontaneously or on slight trauma. It ranges in color from pink to red purple, depending on the age of the lesion.

Young pyogenic granulomas are highly vascular in appearance; older lesions tend to become more collagenized and pink. It is painless and bleeds easily because of its extreme vascularity. Sometimes there is exudation of purulent material, but it is not a characteristic feature despite the suggestive name of the lesion. Some lesions have brown casts if hemorrhage has occurred into the lesion.

Lesions are slightly more common on the maxillary gingiva than the mandibular, anterior areas than posterior areas and on the facial aspect of the gingival than the lingual aspect. Some extend between the teeth and involve both the facial and lingual gingiva. They measure a few millimeters in size to several centimeters in diameter.

Although the pyogenic granuloma can develop at any age, it is most common in children and young adults. Most studies also demonstrate a definite female predilection, possibly because of the vascular effects of female hormones.

Pregnancy Epulis or Pregnancy Tumor

50

Contents

50.1 Histopathologic Features... 214
50.2 Treatment.. 214
Reference... 214

It is a clinical term used to describe a reddish-purple often nodular and ulcerated localized tumor that bleeds easily and may grow rapidly. It is claimed that the clinical onset of most is at about the second or third month of pregnancy, gradually increases in size, and after delivery may or may not regress. It is now believed that "pregnancy tumor" is simply a pyogenic granuloma which occurs as a result of local minor trauma or irritation and in which the reaction is probably intensified by the endocrine alteration occurring during pregnancy. There appears to be no justification to retain the term "pregnancy tumor" since this lesion with an identical clinical and histologic nature is seen in men and in nonpregnant women.

Mills et al. [1] showed a male predilection in children (82%), a female predilection up to the age of 39 years (86%), and no sex predilection in patients more than 39 years of age.

Many authors stress the importance of some form of chronic low-grade irritation (calculus, plaque, restorations) as the initiating factor, with the response enhanced by female sex hormones. The increase in the incidence of occurrence of this tumor during the last two trimesters of pregnancy is related to the steady rise in the placental hormones, namely, the progesterone and estrogen. The resolution of the lesions after the delivery is related to the decline of the placental hormone levels.

Epulis granulomatosis is a term used to describe the hyperplastic growth of granulation tissue that sometimes arises in healing extraction sockets. These lesions resemble pyogenic granulomas and usually represent a granulation tissue reaction to bony sequestra in the socket.

© The Author(s), under exclusive license to Springer Nature Singapore Pte Ltd. 2024
K. Paiwal et al., *Handbook of Oral and Maxillofacial Giant Cell Lesions*,
https://doi.org/10.1007/978-981-97-2863-3_50

50.1 Histopathologic Features

Microscopic examination shows a highly vascular proliferation that resembles granulation tissue. The surface epithelium if present may be atrophic or thin. If it is ulcerated, it shows fibrinous exudates of varying thickness over the epithelium. The most striking feature is the occurrence of a vast number of small and large endothelium-lined vascular channels that are engorged with red blood cells, the extreme proliferation of fibroblasts, and budding endothelial cells. These vessels sometimes are organized in lobular aggregates. A mixed inflammatory cell infiltrate of neutrophils, plasma cells, lymphocytes, and occasional giant cells is evident. The connective tissue stroma is typically delicate, although frequently fasciculi of collagen fibers are noted coursing through the tissue mass. The old mature lesions may sometimes clinically and microscopically resemble a fibroepithelial polyp or even a typical fibroma.

50.2 Treatment

Pyogenic granuloma is treated by surgical excision. Care should be taken to scale the adjacent tooth and make certain that it is free of calculus.

For pregnancy tumor, surgical and periodontal treatment should be completed during the second trimester, with continued surveillance of home care until after delivery. If the lesion does not cause any significant functional or esthetic problems, it should not be excised during pregnancy, as they may recur. Ultimately, they resolve spontaneously after parturition.

Reference

1. https://pubmed.ncbi.nlm.nih.gov/7435775/.

MIX
Papier aus verantwortungsvollen Quellen
Paper from responsible sources
FSC® C105338

If you have any concerns about our products,
you can contact us on
ProductSafety@springernature.com

In case Publisher is established outside the EU,
the EU authorized representative is:
**Springer Nature Customer Service Center GmbH
Europaplatz 3, 69115 Heidelberg, Germany**

Printed by Libri Plureos GmbH
in Hamburg, Germany